LIVING THERAPY SERIES

Person-centred Counselling Supervision

Supervision

Personal and Professional

Richard Bryant-Jefferies

Radcliffe Publishing
Oxford • Seattle

Radcliffe Publishing Ltd
18 Marcham Road
Abingdon
Oxon OX14 1AA
United Kingdom

www.radcliffe-oxford.com
Electronic catalogue and worldwide online ordering facility.

British Library Cataloguing in Publication Data

A catalogue record for this book is available from the British Library.

ISBN 1 85775 704 1

Typeset by Aarontype Ltd, Easton, Bristol
Printed and bound by TJ International Ltd, Padstow, Cornwall

Lori Russell-Chapin

Contents

Foreword

'The expectation that practising counsellors who are members of the British Association for Counselling will have adequate counselling-supervision was first clearly stated in the 1984 version of the BAC's *Code of Ethics and Practice for Counsellors:*

Counsellors monitor their counselling work through regular supervision by professionally competent supervisors ... (p. 2, para. 3.3.)

This view is repeated and elaborated in later versions of the code for counsellors.

It has been my impression, gained from discussions at conferences, that in 1984 this was accepted as an ideal to receive supervision but that a significant number of counsellors were having practical difficulties in obtaining supervision. The position seems to have changed over recent years. Since 1984 not only has (i) supervision come to be viewed as essential to competent practice but also (ii) the understanding of what constitutes supervision has developed in response to an increasing literature on the subject and through shared experience on supervision training courses.' (Bond, 1996, p. 460)

So it was as recent as 20 years ago that supervision became a necessary requirement for membership of the BAC, as it was known in those days. (Although, I realise that for the majority of counsellors today, 20 years seems ages!) I myself had been familiar with 'non-managerial supervision' since the 1970s, when I undertook a training course in non-managerial supervision in the Youth Service at Goldsmith College. The concept of 'non-managerial' supervision, which was concerned with the support and development of the worker in relation to their work, rather than the work itself, sits well with what has become known as person-centred supervision. Emphasis was placed on the relationship between the supervisor and worker, so that the worker would feel confident to bring what they perceived as their weaknesses, failures and fears in their work with often difficult and demanding young people.

I am happy that Richard places so much importance on this element of *relationship* in this book, and that it is apparent in every chapter. It is essential that person-centred counsellors are offered the core conditions themselves, and a trust in their own experiencing of their therapeutic relationships with their clients, a reinforcing of the supervisee's internal locus of evaluation, and the encouragement of the development of a reflective 'self supervisor'. Richard explores the implications of person-centred counsellors having to undergo supervision from other schools of therapy, where the element of collaboration is not at the forefront.

The succinct synopsis of the theory behind person-centred counselling and the personality theory provides a useful backdrop for the scenarios presented in the chapters, and not only does Richard succeed in his aim 'of bringing the experience of supervision alive for the reader', he also manages to relate the theory to practice throughout, in a lively and sometimes provocative manner.

Most of the time, I found myself reading this book as a trainer in person-centred supervision, and would find it useful training material. I agree with Richard that trainees in person-centred counselling training courses could well find it helpful and reassuring when having to find their first supervisor and embark on the daunting exercise of supervision. The important element in person-centred (or supervisee-centred) counselling of non-directiveness is stressed throughout. It is not the intention of person-centred supervisors to tell their supervisees how they should be doing it, or even that they are doing it wrong. Often it is about facilitating the supervisee to know what they know. However, the question of ethics and boundaries is not avoided, and is often discussed under the heading of congruence (both in the supervisor and supervisee).

This book, as the author states, is timely. I am concerned in my own supervisory practice, often of supervisors, to hear of misunderstandings about person-centred supervision. (As indeed there are many misunderstandings about the approach itself.) Issues arising in trainee placements, such as assessment, boundaries, challenge, confrontation, etc. are constantly being raised, and the fact that we might deal differently with these issues in the context of person-centred supervision than in other approaches sometimes causes problems for volunteer coordinators and/or group supervisors, among others. It could be helpful for professionals from other approaches to read this book, to help them understand (and possibly appreciate) our differences. In this book, Richard has brought together examples of supervision sessions in the Living Therapy series, so supervision of trainee counsellors is not specifically included. Next on the list Richard?

Finally, it is so appropriate that Richard has dedicated this book to Tony Merry and I am grateful to be contributing in this small way. In 1991 the IPCL (Institute for Person-Centred Learning) identified a need for person-centred supervisors and Tony and I worked together on the Supervising Person-Centred Practice diploma programme until his death. We were peer supervisors for a number of years, and much of what I know about person-centred supervision I learned from him.

Irene Fairhurst
Client-centred counsellor/psychotherapist
Person-centred supervisor
Consultant and trainer
Co-founder, British Association for the Person-Centred Approach
and Institute for Person-Centred Learning
January 2005

Reference

Bond T (1996) *Counselling Supervision: ethical issues in counselling*. The BAC Counselling Reader. Sage Publications, London.

Preface

Having written a number of books now in the Living Therapy series, each providing a demonstration of the application of the person-centred approach to counselling and psychotherapy to clients presenting with particular issues, it seemed to me time to focus more on the supervisory element of the therapeutic process. Supervision sessions have been included within the person-centred dialogues within the Living Therapy series. I view this as crucial in order to demonstrate counselling or psychotherapy in action. However, it seemed timely to draw from the experience of writing these various titles and produce a volume dedicated specifically to the practice of supervising person-centred counsellors.

I have been further encouraged in this by the publication in 2004 of *Freedom to Practise* by Keith Tudor and Mike Worrall, in which they set out to present a model, and theoretical base, for person-centred supervision. I personally found their ideas, together with those who contributed their own chapters within their book, to be extremely thought-provoking. So I thank them for that. I do not aim to establish such an in-depth theoretical exploration in this book. Rather, I am seeking to convey an experience to the reader, a sense of the process. I want to bring the supervision experience alive to the reader.

In considering person-centred supervision we need to establish that there are two areas of emphasis as follows.

- The supervision presented seeks to demonstrate a person-centred way of working.
- The counsellors being supervised are bringing their experience of working in a person-centred way.

There is not always a coinciding of models between the supervisee and the supervision. Some argue that they should be the same, others that it can be of value to have a contrast in theoretical model. Speaking for myself, I have largely experienced person-centred supervision of my person-centred practice. This has helped me to 'talk my own language', to be able to explore at perhaps greater theoretical depth the processes taking place within the counselling and supervision sessions from the person-centred perspective. However, I have also experienced supervision from a psychodynamic perspective and I found it useful for someone to be offering alternative angles on process and content.

I have also experienced supervising counsellors who apply a different theoretical model to their practice of the person-centred approach. Again, I have found this valuable and stimulating, and thought-provoking for my supervisees. However, I would also like to comment that perhaps my most challenging group to work with were those pursuing an integrative approach, as so often what I found was a student counsellor not being trained to theoretical depth for any particular approach and who therefore struggled to establish a genuine core model. Person-centred working might then become another 'tool' or 'technique' to apply to clients with particular issues, or perhaps be seen as the basic relational framework on which other ways of working were then constructed, with little awareness that at the heart of the person-centred approach lies the tenet that the six conditions for constructive personality change are not only necessary, but more to the point, are sufficient.

So I would say that when someone is beginning their career as a counsellor, and particularly whilst they are still training, having a supervisor working to the theoretical model that the counsellor is seeking to apply seems to me to be extremely important. I have supervised trainees and discussed this with them, particularly those who have been attending integrative training and may have periods of training specific to particular theoretical approaches with the risk that their clients become guinea pigs on which to 'try out' the latest bit of theory or technique learned in the classroom. As a counsellor gains in experience and more fully internalises their practice from a particular theoretical perspective, then they may well find supervision from an alternative model challenging and enriching.

In *Person-Centred Counselling Supervision: personal and professional*, I have brought together examples of supervision sessions from the Living Therapy titles, and have sought to present each one as an example of person-centred supervisory practice of person-centred counselling. The supervision sessions deal with a range of issues that arise when working with clients who are seeking counselling in order to resolve difficulties from the following range of difficult human experience:

- problematic alcohol use
- stress, in the time-limited context of a GP surgery
- sexual abuse
- drug use
- bullying at school
- temptation to use drugs in teenage years
- faced with a diagnosis of progressive disability
- coming to terms with acceptance of the need to use a wheelchair
- breaking free from the effect of a critical and rejecting parent
- coping with a son with a mental health and substance use problem
- struggling to resolve psychotic symptoms linked to traumatic early life experiences and later cannabis use.

Each supervision session is introduced with a summary of the background to what has occurred in the previous counselling sessions and, where they have occurred, previous supervision sessions. Points for discussion are then included at the end of each chapter to stimulate further thought and debate on issues linked to the supervision dialogue. Reflections from the supervisor are contained within the dialogue. Comment boxes containing text that discusses the supervisory process that is occurring through the supervisor's reflections appear throughout the chapters. I have noted how, when reviewing the supervisory process some months on from writing, different themes have struck me, and I can see interactions within the dialogues having fresh meanings. I am perhaps more detached now from the creative process of writing and from this perspective can recognise more clearly elements of the supervisory process as being deserving of further comment.

I want to make clear that this book does not attempt to demonstrate some kind of definitive way to apply person-centred principles to supervision. All supervisors have their own style, developed over their years of experience. But I hope to demonstrate core principles. There are times when the supervisors lose their person-centred focus and are themselves needing to take their work to supervision to explore issues that arise. Nevertheless, I hope that this compilation of supervision sessions offers a perspective through fictitious examples of how the attitudinal qualities of congruence, unconditional positive regard and empathic understanding play a part in supporting a supervisee in his or her work with a client.

I hope too that it will prove valuable to experienced and novice supervisors, and to those uncertain about supervising counsellors working in areas outside their own professional experience. I have often heard, for instance, counsellors saying that they cannot take particular issues to a supervisor because they do not work with that issue – drug abuse and alcohol problems are two that come to mind, and also counselling young people and people who have been targets of sexual abuse.

I hope that this book will be read widely by counsellors in training who are preparing to be supervised. How a counsellor uses supervision is important. What do you bring? What can you expect? Will the supervisor 'tell me off'? For me, the supervisor may bring greater experience into the collaborative process of supervision, but they are not necessarily the only 'expert' in the room. I will say a little more in the introduction about collaborative supervision which I believe captures the essence of what a person-centred supervisor is seeking to achieve with their supervisee.

Richard Bryant-Jefferies
January 2005

About the author

Richard Bryant-Jefferies qualified as a person-centred counsellor/therapist in 1994 and remains passionate about the application and effectiveness of this approach. Between early 1995 and mid-2003 Richard worked at a community drug and alcohol service in Surrey, though more recently he has been appointed to manage NHS substance misuse services in the Royal Borough of Kensington and Chelsea in London, part of the Central and North West London Mental Health NHS Trust. He has experience of offering counselling and supervision in NHS, GP and private settings, and has provided training through 'alcohol awareness and response' workshops.

He also offers workshops based on the use of written dialogue as a contribution to continuing professional development and within training programmes. See www.bryant-jefferies.freeserve.co.uk.

Richard had his first book on a counselling theme published in 2001, *Counselling the Person Beyond the Alcohol Problem* (Jessica Kingsley Publishers), providing theoretical yet practical insights into the application of the person-centred approach within the context of the 'cycle of change' model that has been widely adopted to describe the process of change in the field of addiction. Since then he has been writing for the ongoing Living Therapy book series, producing the titles on person-centred dialogues of *Problem Drinking, Time Limited Therapy in Primary Care, Counselling a Survivor of Child Sexual Abuse, Counselling a Recovering Drug User, Counselling Young People, Counselling for Progressive Disability, Relationship Counselling: Sons and Their Mothers, Responding to a Serious Mental Health Problem.* The aim of the series is to bring the reader a direct experience of the counselling process, an exposure to the thoughts and feelings of both client and counsellor as they encounter each other on the therapeutic journey, and an insight into the value and importance of supervision.

Richard is keen to bring the experience of the therapeutic process, from the standpoint and application of the person-centred approach, to a wider audience. He is convinced that the principles and attitudinal values of this approach and the emphasis it places on the therapeutic relationship are key to helping people create greater authenticity in themselves and in their lives, leading to a fuller and more satisfying human experience. By writing fictional accounts to try and bring the therapeutic process alive, to help readers engage with the characters within the narrative – client, counsellor and supervisor – he hopes to take the reader on a journey into the counselling room. Whether we think of it as pulling back the curtains or opening a door, it is about enabling people to access what can and does occur within the therapeutic process.

In this latest volume he draws from supervision sessions within the series in order to focus a similar searchlight specifically into the supervision room, to shed light upon the supervisory process from the angle of person-centred practice.

Acknowledgements

I would like to thank my various supervisors over the years, and my supervisees, for the learning they have given me and which, I am sure, in different ways, has influenced the content of this book. I would particularly like to thank Irene Fairhurst and Tony Merry, my trainers in supervising person-centred practice. Their experience and enthusiasm for the approach made a huge difference to my life. Irene, thank you for the Foreword. It has meant a lot to me to have you write this given how much you were involved in my person-centred training over the years. And Tony, who sadly died in 2004, I will be forever grateful for your great contribution to my learning to practice person-centredness.

I would also, once again, like to thank the editorial and production team at Radcliffe Publishing, and encourage any reader who has an idea for a book on some area of person-centred counselling and psychotherapy to contact them.

Dedication

I wish to dedicate this book to Tony Merry. Tony died on 22nd August 2004. It was a shock to me, and to so many others whose lives were touched by his presence. He was one of my trainers when I began my initial training in person-centred practice, and for my training in person-centred supervision. I have many clear memories of Tony during those days of learning: his humour, his wisdom, his passion for the approach, and a constant sense that when Tony was in the room something was going to happen. It usually did!

Tony was a co-founder of BAPCA (British Association for the Person Centred Approach) and long time editor of *Person Centred Practice*. A significant and respected author in his own right, he had recently been appointed Reader at the University of East London. On 22nd August 2004 the world was robbed of a person who was so alive to the person-centred approach, whose writings and words had touched so many people, and who still had so much more to offer.

Introduction

The need for an appreciation and understanding of the nature and purpose of the supervisory relationship is vital for both counsellor and supervisor. It is not a therapeutic relationship and yet it has strong therapeutic value. It is supportive, it has a certain collegial nature to it, a meeting of co-professionals to explore the impact that a relationship with a client is having on a supervisee, and of clarifying, as well, the ongoing, developing supervisor–supervisee relationship in order to ensure that the counselling work can be explored openly, freely and transparently.

Many professions do not recognise the need for some form of personal and process supervision, and often what is offered is line management. However, it is the norm for all professionals working in the healthcare and social care environment in this age of regulation to be formally accredited or registered and to work to their own professional organisation's code of ethics or practice. For instance, counselling practitioners registered with the British Association for Counselling and Psychotherapy are required to have regular supervision and continuing professional development to maintain registration. Counsellors are required to receive regular supervision in order to explore the dynamics of the relationship with the client, the impact of the work on the counsellor and on the client, to receive support, and to provide an opportunity for an experienced co-professional to monitor the supervisee's work in relation to ethical standards and codes of practice.

The publication *Research on Supervision of Counsellors and Psychotherapists: a systematic scoping search* (Wheeler, 2003) draws together a wide range of research findings into many aspects of supervision, not only of counsellors and psychotherapists, but amongst other professions as well. There are many quotations and references and it would not do it justice to mention one or two. However, I was disappointed to find it difficult to ascertain whether the research papers drawn on were specific to a particular approach. In some cases this could be surmised from the language used, but I was not able to draw anything specific linked to person-centred supervision, though I may have missed it. Either way, it indicates to me the need for more research, and more awareness of research, into the practice and effectiveness of the person-centred model of supervision.

Whilst professionals other than counsellors will gain much from this book in helping them understand the value of a person-centred approach to supervision, it is essential that they follow the standards, safeguards and ethical codes of their own professional organisation, and are appropriately trained and supervised to work with them on the issues that arise. It is also hoped that readers from other professions recognise the value of some form of supportive and collaborative supervision in order to help them become more authentically present with their own clients.

Before exploring the nature of person-centred supervision, it might be helpful to draw together key components of the person-centred approach to counselling, particularly for those readers who, whilst interested in the practice of supervision, are new to the theory behind person-centred working. The following section describes some of the essentials of the person-centred approach to counselling and psychotherapy.

The person-centred approach to counselling

It is worth saying something at this point about the essence of the person-centred approach (PCA), particularly as the approach when applied in a therapeutic setting is often referred to as 'client-centred therapy'. Although not everyone regards the terms as interchangeable, and prefers to maintain this classical differentiation, I have used the term 'person-centred approach' in the Living Therapy series as I personally prefer the idea of emphasising the client as a person – their personhood, if you like – rather than their role in the therapeutic relationship as 'the client'.

The person-centred approach was formulated by Carl Rogers, and references are made to his ideas within the text of the book. However, it will be helpful for readers who are unfamiliar with this way of working to have an appreciation of its theoretical base.

Rogers proposed that certain conditions, when present within a therapeutic relationship, would enable the client to develop towards what he termed 'fuller functionality'. Over a number of years he refined these ideas, which he defined as 'the necessary and sufficient conditions for constructive personality change'. These he described as follows.

1 Two persons are in psychological contact.
2 The first, whom we shall term the client, is in a state of incongruence, being vulnerable or anxious.
3 The second person, whom we shall term the therapist, is congruent or integrated in the relationship.
4 The therapist experiences unconditional positive regard for the client.
5 The therapist experiences an empathic understanding of the client's internal frame of reference and endeavours to communicate this experience to the client.
6 The communication to the client of the therapist's empathic understanding and unconditional positive regard is to a minimal degree achieved. (Rogers, 1957, p. 96)

The first necessary and sufficient condition given for constructive personality change is that of 'two persons being in psychological contact'. However, although he later published this as simply 'contact' (Rogers, 1959) it is suggested (Wyatt and Sanders, 2002, p. 6) that this was actually written in 1953–4. They quote Rogers as defining contact in the following terms: 'Two persons are in psychological contact, or have the minimum essential relationship when each makes a perceived or subceived difference in the experiential field of the other' (Rogers, 1959, p. 207). A recent exploration of the nature of psychological contact from a person-centred perspective is given by Warner (2002).

Rogers defined empathy as meaning 'entering the private perceptual world of the other . . . being sensitive, moment by moment, to the changing felt meanings which flow in this other person . . . It means sensing meanings of which he or she is scarcely aware, but not trying to uncover totally unconscious feelings' (Rogers, 1980, p. 142). It is a very delicate process, and it provides, I believe, a foundation block. The counsellor's role is primarily to establish empathic rapport and communicate empathic understanding to the client.

Within this relationship the counsellor seeks to maintain an attitude of unconditional positive regard towards the client and all that they disclose. This is not 'agreeing with', it is simply warm acceptance. Rogers writes, 'when the therapist is experiencing a positive, acceptant attitude towards whatever the client *is* at that moment, therapeutic movement or change is more likely to occur' (Rogers, 1980, p. 116). Mearns and Thorne suggest that 'unconditional positive regard is the label given to the fundamental attitude of the person-centred counsellor towards her client. The counsellor who holds this attitude deeply values the humanity of her client and is not deflected in that valuing by any particular client behaviours. The attitude manifests itself in the counsellor's consistent acceptance of and enduring warmth towards her client' (Mearns and Thorne, 1988, p. 59).

Last, but by no means least, is that state of being that Rogers referred to as congruence, but which has also been described in terms of 'realness', 'transparency', 'genuineness', 'authenticity'. Indeed Rogers wrote that '. . . genuineness, realness or congruence . . . this means that the therapist is openly being the feelings and attitudes that are flowing within at the moment . . . the term transparent catches the flavour of this condition' (Rogers, 1980, p. 115). Putting this into the therapeutic setting, we can say that 'congruence is the state of being of the counsellor when her outward responses to her client consistently match the inner feelings and sensations which she has in relation to her client' (Mearns and Thorne, 1999, p. 84). Haugh interestingly explores the confusion over the language associated with congruence and concludes that 'congruence . . . is a state of being' and that 'in the being they will be experienced as the outcomes of congruence – authentic, genuine, transparent and real' (Haugh, 1998, p. 49).

I would suggest that any congruent expression by the counsellor of their feelings or reactions has to emerge through the process of being in a therapeutic relationship with the client. It is a disciplined response and not an open door to endless self-disclosure. Congruent expression is perhaps most appropriate and therapeutically valuable where it is informed by the existence of an empathic understanding of the client's inner world, and is offered in a climate of a genuine warm acceptance towards the client.

It is my belief that by offering someone a non-judgemental, warm and accepting, and authentic relationship – in truth an experience of love (perhaps we need to speak more of therapeutic love) – then that person can grow into a fresh sense of self in which their potential as a person can become more fulfilled. Such an experience fosters an opportunity for the client to redefine themselves as they experience the presence of the therapist's congruence, empathy and unconditional positive regard. This process can take time. Often the personality change that is required to sustain a shift away from what have been termed 'conditions of worth' requires a lengthy period of therapeutic work, bearing in mind that the person may be struggling to unravel a sense of self that has been developed, sustained and reinforced for many decades of life.

The term 'conditions of worth' applies to the conditioning that is frequently present in childhood, and at other times in life, when a person experiences that their worth is conditional on their doing something, or behaving, in a certain way. This is usually to satisfy someone else's needs, and can be contrary to the client's own sense of what would be a satisfying experience. The values of others become a feature of the individual's structure of self. The person moves away from being true to themselves, learning instead to remain 'true' to their conditioned sense of worth. This state of being in the client is challenged by the person-centred therapist by offering them unconditional positive regard and warm acceptance. Such a therapist, by genuinely offering these therapeutic attitudes, provides the client with an opportunity to be exposed to what may be a new experience or one that in the past they have dismissed, preferring to stay with that which matches and therefore reinforces their conditioned sense of worth and sense of self. Unconditional positive regard and warm acceptance offered consistently over time can, and do, enable clients to begin to question their beliefs about themselves and to begin to build into their structure of self the capacity to see and experience themselves as being of value for who they are. It enables them to liberate themselves from the constraints of patterns of conditioning.

A crucial feature or factor in this process is the presence of what Rogers termed 'the actualising tendency'; a tendency towards fuller and more complete personhood with an associated greater fulfilment of their potentialities. The role of the person-centred counsellor is to provide the facilitative climate within which this tendency can work constructively. The 'therapist trusts the actualizing tendency of the client and truly believes that the client who experiences the freedom of a fostering psychological climate will resolve his or her own problems' (Bozarth, 1998, p. 4). This is fundamental to the application of the person-centred approach. Rogers (1986, p. 198) writes: 'the person-centred approach is built on a basic trust in the person ... (It) depends on the actualizing tendency present in every living organism – the tendency to grow, to develop, to realize its full potential. This way of being trusts the constructive directional flow of the human being towards a more complex and complete development. It is this directional flow that we aim to release.'

From this theoretical perspective we can argue that the person-centred counsellor's role is essentially facilitative. The presence of a diagnosis becomes secondary to the simple fact that the client is attending with some degree of psychological discomfort that is manifesting through a set of symptoms and behaviours that have been diagnostically labelled as a specific 'illness'. Creating the therapeutic climate of empathic understanding, unconditional positive regard and authenticity creates a relational climate in which the client's own inherent capacity towards actualising their fuller potential as a person can become directed towards establishing a fresh sense of self that is liberated from the 'conditions of worth' perhaps rooted in traumatising experiences that are all too often at the root of psychological discomfort.

Whilst it is recognised that there will be certain conditions of mind which will require chemical interventions because the condition is the result of chemical imbalance or organic deficiencies, we should not allow this to blind us to the possibility that there are underlying environmental and experiential factors that have had a major contribution to a person's state of mind and emotion. I describe it thus because whilst emphasis is on 'mental health', it is important to keep visible the fact that for many people their difficulties and psychological discomforts are strongly linked to difficult emotional experiencing. It is important to acknowledge that symptomology might be better seen as a kind of experiential flashing neon sign, drawing attention to the fact that something is wrong. If our treatment responses are simply concerned with turning off the flashing light because it is a problem to us, rather than seeking the underlying reason for which it is flashing, then we have a system that goes no further than symptom management. Whilst this may well have a part to play in bringing a client symptom relief, it should not be confused with treatment of the underlying cause.

In addressing these factors the therapeutic relationship is central. A therapeutic approach, such as person-centred, affirms that it is not what you do so much as how you are with your client that is therapeutically significant, and this 'how you are' has to be received by the client. Gaylin (2001, p. 103) highlights the importance of client perception. 'If clients believe that their therapist is working on their behalf – if they perceive caring and understanding – then therapy is likely to be successful. It is the condition of attachment and the perception of connection that have the power to release the faltered actualization of the self.' He goes on to stress how 'we all need to feel connected, prized – loved', describing human beings as 'a species born into mutual interdependence', and that there 'can be no self outside the context of others. Loneliness is dehumanizing and isolation anathema to the human condition. The relationship,' he suggests 'is what psychotherapy is all about.'

In a previous volume in this series I used the analogy of treating a wilting plant (Bryant-Jefferies, 2003, p. 12). We can spray it with some specific herbicide or pesticide to eradicate a perceived disease that may be present in the plant, and that may be enough. But perhaps the true cause of the disease is that the plant is located in harsh surroundings, perhaps too much sun and not enough water, poor soil, near other plants that it finds it difficult to survive near. Maybe by offering the plant a healthier environment that will facilitate greater nourishment according to the needs of the plant, it may reach its potential to become a strong, healthy plant. Yes, the chemical intervention may also be helpful, but if the true causes of the diseases are environmental – essentially the plant's relationship with that which surrounds it – then it won't actually achieve sustainable growth. We may not be able to transplant it, but we can provide water, nutrients and maybe shade from a fierce sun. Therapy, it seems to me, exists to provide this healthy environment within which the wilting client can begin the process of receiving the nourishment (in the form of healthy relational experience) that can enable them, in time, to become a more fully functioning person.

There is currently growing interest in, and much debate about, theoretical developments within the person-centred world and its application. Discussions on the theme of Rogers' therapeutic conditions presented by various key members of the person-centred community have been published (Bozarth and Wilkins, 2001; Haugh and Merry, 2001; Wyatt, 2001; Wyatt and Sanders, 2002). Mearns and Thorne have recently produced a timely publication revising and developing key aspects of person-centred theory (2000). Wilkins has produced a book that addresses most effectively many of the criticisms levelled against person-centred working (2003). It seems to me that the relational component of the person-centred approach, based on the presence of the core conditions, is emerging strongly as a counter to the sense of isolation that frequently accompanies deep psychological and emotional problems, and which is a feature of materialistic societies as we enter the 21st century.

This is obviously a very brief introduction to the approach. Person-centred theory continues to develop as practitioners and theoreticians consider its application in various fields of therapeutic work and extend our theoretical understanding of developmental and therapeutic processes. At times it feels like it has become more than just individuals, rather it feels like a group of colleagues, based around the world, working together to penetrate deeper towards a more complete theory of the human condition. Person-centred or client-centred theory and practice has a key role in this process. It is an exciting time.

A person-centred approach to supervision

Merry (2002, pp. 170–1) has pointed out that 'little has been written about person-centred supervision'. He cites some examples of written material in this area, for instance Mearns (1997), Hackney and Goodyear (1984), Patterson (1997), Worral (2001) and Merry (2001). References have also been made to person-centred supervision in other titles (Mearns and Thorne, 1999; Patterson, 2000) and more recently Tudor and Worrall (2004) have drawn together a number of theoretical and experiential strands from within and outside of the person-centred tradition in order to develop a theoretical position on the person-centred approach to supervision.

In my view, this latter publication is particularly timely, defining the necessary factors for effective supervision within this way of working, and the respective responsibilities of both supervisor and supervisee in keeping with person-centred values and principles. They contrast person-centred working with other approaches to supervision and emphasise the importance of the therapeutic space as a place within which practitioners 'can dialogue freely between their personal philosophy and the philosophical assumptions which underlie their chosen theoretical orientation' (Tudor and Worrall, 2004, pp. 94–5). They affirm the values and attitudes of person-centred working and explore their application to the supervisory relationship, in particular the six necessary and sufficient conditions for constructive personality change in the context of supervision (Tudor and Worrall, 2004). They question whether they are all indeed necessary and sufficient for effective supervision.

Is the purpose of supervision to bring about 'constructive personality change' in the supervisee? Well, this may be a product of the supervisory relationship, however, I would question whether this is the primary emphasis. The supervisee comes to supervision in order to ensure that he or she is able to function effectively as a counsellor. Supervision offers the opportunity to acknowledge difficulties and weaknesses, and to celebrate and value strengths and achievements. It is a place in which the supervisee can honestly and openly ask questions of his or her practice and abilities, and process what emerges, or has emerged, into awareness.

For this to occur, it seems to me reasonable that there must be some degree of psychological contact. Tudor and Worrall (2004) indicate their view that supervision by email is possible but that it does not require psychological contact. But if we take the view that psychological contact means that the presence of one person affects another in some way, then surely this presence is being communicated via email. Do you actually have to have moment-to-moment communication for psychological contact to occur? Can it be, as with email, time-delayed and still be considered to carry a form of psychological contact? I disagree with Tudor and Worrall who argue that this first condition is not necessary for supervision. I think psychological contact is required for effective supervision but, as typified by email, what we need to do is broaden our definition of psychological contact.

Whether the supervisee needs to be in a state of incongruence for effective supervision to occur is in my view much more questionable. Tudor and Worrall argue that this second condition is not strictly necessary for the process of supervision. Supervisees may well be quite congruent but still find value in exploring themes and issues that have arisen within their counselling work.

I do believe in the importance of the supervisor being in a state of congruence, not only in the sense of their own experience, awareness and communication, but also in terms of their role as a supervisor. This means owning the responsibilities that come with this role. Not that the supervisor is responsible *for* the supervisee, or for their client, but they do have a responsibility *to* their supervisee and, through them, to the clients that the supervisee is working with.

I also consider unconditional positive regard to be an important feature of the effective supervisory relationship. It is no good offering a conditional attitude if you wish to encourage a free and open exploration. The supervisor is not some Victorian teacher, ready to strike fear into the heart of a pupil who makes a mistake or choose a line of thought that differs from the accepted norm. The person-centred supervisor will want to feel warm acceptance of their clients and their work and, yes, if they feel uncomfortable about the quality of practice, will raise this, but in a way that will hopefully encourage the supervisee to explore and develop their own responses and solutions.

Empathy, too, is a necessary condition for the emergence of an effective supervisory relationship. As a supervisee I would certainly want to know that my supervisor is seeking to understand my experience and my process as I wrestle with some facet of my counselling work.

Finally, there is the need for what is present to be communicated by the supervisor, and for that communication to be accurately received by the supervisee. Yes, again, a necessary factor in the creation and maintenance of an effective supervisory relationship. So, what we are considering are the necessary and sufficient conditions for a constructive supervisory relationship. And to me this does not necessarily require incongruence in the supervisee, but it does require the other five conditions.

Worrall (2001) has emphasised the particular role of empathy, and Merry (2001) the significance of congruence in supervision. I would conclude that what is necessary are those ways of being of the supervisor which enable a supervisee to become openly present in the supervisory relationship without experiencing a need to screen out uncomfortable experiences linked to their counselling (and supervision) work. In terms of person-centred theory, these necessary conditions, so long as they can encourage the openness and spirit of collaborative exploration, will be deemed sufficient.

The following seems to me to be a very simple (but by no means simplistic) definition of person-centred supervision: 'person-centred supervision is concerned with how you, the counsellor, form relationships with your clients, and how you can deepen your empathic understanding of them whilst remaining as congruent as you can and experiencing unconditional positive regard towards them' (Merry, 2002, p. 170). In other words, person-centred supervision is concerned with ensuring that the counsellor is offering, or able to offer, the attitudinal qualities and values that are the essence of the person-centred approach.

The supervisory relationship, at least from a person-centred theoretical framework, has to be of a collaborative nature, which I have described in terms of being a process of 'collaborative review' in previous books in the Living Therapy series. Supervision provides a process of reviewing not only the content of counselling sessions, but also the processes that emerge in order to ensure that the counsellor can offer, in line with what Merry indicates, a congruent presence, empathic understanding and an experience of unconditional positive regard.

Merry (2002, p. 173) describes what he terms 'collaborative inquiry' as a 'form of research or inquiry in which two people (the supervisor and the counsellor) collaborate or cooperate in an effort to understand what is going on within the counselling relationship and within the counsellor'. He highlights how this 'moves the emphasis away from "doing things right or wrong" (which seems to be the case in some approaches to supervision) to "how is the counsellor *being*, and how is that way of being contributing to the development of a counselling relationship based on the core conditions"'.

For this to occur effectively, the factor of the relationship between supervisor and supervisee has to be recognised as a significant factor. A spirit of openness is vital. It has to be free of any sense of threat so that the supervisee is less likely to screen out material as a result of defensiveness. Merry describes the 'major function of person-centred supervision' as providing 'opportunities for supervisees (counsellors) to experience a relationship that is free of threat, and is supportive and understanding so that they can explore non-defensively what the counselling process means to them, and how they experience themselves in relationship with their clients' (Merry, 2002, p. 173).

Supervision is often about exploring the uncomfortable, the uncertain. Sommerbeck describes it in the following terms. 'Time and again, the therapist will want a place of his own where he feels safe to explore, for example, troubling, albeit unclear, feelings of not being fully congruent in his relationship with a client.' She adds that 'no therapist, however competent or experienced, can avoid getting into situations where he feels uncomfortable with a client . . .' (Sommerbeck, 2003, p. 132). The supervisory relationship offers this space and the opportunity for open and honest exploration.

Merry also adds that 'the collaborative inquiry model views both supervisor and supervisee as equally influential in the search for meaning' (Merry, 2002, p. 188). This equalising of the importance of both participants within the supervisory relationship is, I believe, a significant feature of a person-centred approach to supervision. The intention on the part of the person-centred supervisor will be to offer a relational climate in which the supervisee will feel free to bring material from the counselling sessions, and this will be encouraged not only by a sense of the supervisor's warm acceptance of them as a person, but also by the supervisor's transparent willingness to accept and value the views of the supervisee. In an exploration of a session of counselling, or perhaps a particular response within a session, the striving for meaning and understanding is a collaborative one. Indeed, insight often emerges through the process of interaction and communication, leading supervisor and supervisee to insights and understandings that neither might have reached on their own.

The relational values and attitudes of the person-centred supervisor need, of course, to be experienced by the supervisee. It is as a result of the supportive climate that is engendered through the presence of the attitudes and values of person-centred working that the supervisee is enabled and encouraged to be open both in their expression and communication, and also to their own inner promptings and understandings of the counselling process. For me, supervision is an opportunity for ideas to come alive, for purposeful exploration and yet with that certain openness that welcomes spontaneity as a sudden insight breaks into conscious awareness, often subtle at first yet with appropriate support can begin to be grasped to bring a fuller understanding and appreciation of the counselling experience – and the supervisory experience as well.

Within the supervisory process the supervisor will also need to affirm ethical principles and codes of practice. The supervisor maintains a level of responsibility (as does the supervisee) in ensuring that professional practice does not harm the wellbeing of the client. A person-centred supervisor may experience concerns over a supervisee's practice and will want to draw attention to this. Congruent concern does need to be raised, but it can be done in such a way as to encourage the supervisee to own the difficulty and realise, for themselves, the need for further exploration. In addressing the subject of challenging supervisees, Mearns and Thorne (2000) quote Kilborn: 'supervisees not only need to feel understood and accepted, they also need to know where the supervisor stands ... Challenge within a supervisory relationship is accepted by supervisees, indeed it can be experienced as stimulating and enriching' (Kilborn, 1999, p. 89).

One key area of debate insofar as supervision is concerned is whether a counsellor should receive supervision from someone who works to a similar theoretical model in supervision. As mentioned in the preface, I believe this is important, particularly for trainees who are themselves establishing their own core model of working. Matarazzo and Patterson (1986, p. 838) write that 'it appears important for supervisor and supervisee to have a similar theoretical orientation'. Patterson himself later writes, and emphasises the clarity of his thinking, that 'it is not simply desirable or important, but necessary that the supervisor and supervisee be committed to a theory – and the same theory' (Patterson, 2000, p. 194).

A key aspect of person-centred working is the factor of non-directiveness and, as the name given to practice indicates, that it should indeed be person- or client-centred. Insofar as supervision is concerned, we are therefore talking about the supervision session being 'supervisee-centred', and perhaps this should be coined as the theoretical title of the person- or client-centred approach as applied to the supervisory relationship – 'supervisee-centred supervision'. Patterson (2000, p. 206) draws attention to how 'the supervisor, in respecting the supervisee, allows the supervisee to direct the sessions by selecting and presenting the materials to be considered by the supervisor'.

Merry (2002, p. 196) emphasises the non-directive nature of person-centred supervision, commenting that 'the non-directive attitude of the person-centred supervisor is also a critical factor in determining the outcome of supervision'. In relation to the theme of supervision as an 'heuristic research inquiry', which he explores as a methodology to inform the supervisory process, he writes that the agenda for supervision needs 'to be generally under the control of the supervisee. If the agenda is under external control, by the supervisor or by institutional or professional demands, for example, it is unlikely that the supervisee will be able to connect at a deep level with the issue under consideration. In heuristic terms, immersion of the supervisee's whole self will be compromised, and heuristic self enquiry will not proceed.'

Mearns and Thorne emphasise the individual nature of movement in person-centred counselling, of how uncertain and erratic the process can be. They point out that the counsellor's 'faith in the process' can help sustain them 'through such uncertainty', that the person-centred counsellor trusts the consistent offering of the therapeutic conditions as fully as possible, that movement will occur and that 'the overall direction and effect will be positive' – however erratic or stuck the process might seem at times. Having made these points they then comment that 'this is one reason why inexperienced person-centred counsellors need to be supervised by practitioners from the same tradition, for it can sometimes be difficult to trust the process when it has all the appearance of having ground to a halt. A supervisor from another school of thought might inappropriately panic and encourage the counsellor to push the client at precisely the wrong juncture' (Mearns and Thorne, 1999, p. 148).

The supervision sessions within this volume offer the reader insight into the nature of therapeutic supervision from a person-centred theoretical perspective. For many trainee counsellors, the use of supervision can be something of a mystery, and it is hoped that this book will go a long way to unravelling this. I seek to demonstrate the application of the person-centred supervisory relationship, not that the fictitious supervisors are somehow perfect examples of person-centred practice, for I also seek to include examples of where the supervisory practice becomes problematic. The questions for discussion and reflection at the end of each chapter focus the reader on key issues and provide a framework for reflection and debate. How do the principles of person- or client-centred counselling become translated into supervision practice? The reader will no doubt wish to reflect on their own experience of supervision, either as a supervisee or as a supervisor. Would they have responded differently as the supervisor to the issues presented, or might they, as the client, choose to present their issues differently and thereby, perhaps, seek a different outcome?

Person-centred supervision for other professions and professionals

I have been concerned that whilst the need for supervision is recognised in counselling and psychotherapy, this is not the case in many other fields of therapeutic relationship, such as complementary therapy and other forms of healing where relational factors can have a significant contribution to the healing process. This is also true in medical settings – general practitioners (GPs), for instance. The practitioner–client relationship is important in all forms of treatment/healing/ medical intervention. A GP will emphasise the importance of the relationships they have with their patients, that mutual trust and respect are crucial elements in this. Supervision can help ensure that this relationship is maintained, and where it is damaged in some way, the reasons can be openly explored and steps can be taken to resolve underlying issues.

In his foreword to *Counselling a Recovering Drug User*, Peter Robinson (a GP) writes the following.

> Another important part of the process is that of supervision of the therapist. The reader will not only see that supervision is a desirable facility for a healthworker but is an essential element in supporting the worker and encouraging critical analysis and thus deeper understanding of the relationship and the dynamics of the encounter. Having worked as a doctor for 22 years without ever receiving any formal supervision, after reading this book I feel slightly lacking and quite let down as the benefits are shown so eloquently

in this book, not only for the therapist, but also for the therapeutic process itself. (Bryant-Jefferies, 2003, p. v)

Supervision has relevance as well with psychiatric practice. Rachel Freeth, herself a psychiatric doctor, has written about her experience of having a person-centred supervisor. Working in the NHS within the psychiatric profession brings her many challenges. She writes of the importance of the 'supportive function of supervision' which, she writes of as being in general to be 'alarmingly lacking' in NHS healthcare settings. She uses an interesting analogy, offered to her by her supervisor, in the following terms.

> Working in the NHS and within the mental health profession can sometimes feel like attempting 12 rounds in a boxing ring. This analogy was offered to me recently by my supervisor and I have elaborated on it. He has become my 'second', the person who waits in the corner of the ring, provides me with refreshment, dries me down with a towel, offers me a bucket to spit in, and gives me vital words of support and encouragement. (Freeth, 2004, p. 262)

We can extend this to other areas of medicine. Nurses may have clinical supervision, but it may not always include scope for personal exploration – there may not be time, or the culture may not encourage this. A nurse that I supervised made the comment that, for her, 'supervision was like taking an aspirin for a headache'. It communicated to me the sense of stress build-up and overload, and of the role of supervision in providing a safe and supportive space in which to process and let go.

In the homeopathic profession in the UK, 'supervision is established at student level, mandatory at practitioner registration level, and is an expectation post-registration' (Townsend, 2004, p. 236). Townsend goes on to suggest that 'the person-centred approach comes closest to representing what homeopathic practitioners do when they are with their clients, and thus offers the most consistent model for supervision practice' (Townsend, 2004, pp. 237–8). Supervision is surely about encouraging effective practice, whatever that practice might be. Townsend comments that, 'in homeopathic terms, the question we hold as our focus becomes this: "How can we work together to ensure the supervisee becomes the best homeopath she can be?" The function of the supervisor is to create the atmosphere that will enable the student to find his or her own style of being a homeopath, by adhering to the person-centre ideal of offering the necessary and sufficient conditions, even in the face of the supervisee who appeals for help or who asks for instructions' (Townsend, 2004, pp. 238–9).

As well as improving the quality of a practitioner's professional work, supervision also contributes to personal growth and to clarifying and clearing the impact that clients can have on our psychological wellbeing. Whatever our professional discipline, we will be affected to some degree by our clients. We can carry this effect into our work with our next client, or into our family and friendships. We can also experience the reverse, bringing tensions from outside into our relationship with clients, some of which we may not even be aware of.

A client or patient discloses that he has a difficulty with crowds, 'I feel so shaky and uncomfortable, I want to run and hide'. Oh no, the practitioner thinks, as he realises that's how he has been feeling. He realises the client is looking at him, he's stopped talking; the practitioner has stopped listening. 'Sorry', he says, 'please continue'. The practitioner puts on a smile but is shaken and it persists after the client has left. The client leaves feeling more unsettled and never comes back for a further appointment. In any helping relationship the practitioner is touched by the inner world of the client. As a result of this psychological contact, unresolved elements within the practitioner's emotional and mental nature can become blocks to the client's therapeutic process by obstructing the flow of congruence and accurate empathic understanding. The practitioner's reactions can discourage the client's self-healing potential – and in extreme cases may add to a client's psychological damage.

A kind of resonance is established in which the whole region of discomfort becomes more than the sum of the two parts (people) being brought into the relationship. Unravelling these blocks or resonances can ensure that the practitioner–client relationship can continue to develop in a psychologically healthy manner. It may also help to ensure that clients no longer mysteriously stop attending.

The practitioner may at times feel stuck with a 'something' that is very real and present yet somehow cannot be defined; a kind of sense that something is going on yet it cannot quite be grasped and verbalised. 'There's something I'm left feeling after seeing this client but I can't get a hold on it.' This is not unusual and the acknowledgement of the presence of the 'something' in collaboration with the supervisor can help to clarify it, which in turn can inform practice and have a beneficial knock-on effect with the client. Sometimes these 'somethings' can be quite profound and can be linked to pre-verbal experiences in the client (or the supervisor), or to material that exists right on the edge of awareness.

Within the supervisory process there may be times when it is necessary to explore clusters of issues, when a theme seems to run through a number of clients. Is this a theme that is coincidentally present, or is it a 'something' present within the practitioner that is getting caught up in the relational dynamics? It may simply be that clients came along with similar issues and so the need is to work on ensuring some degree of differentiation. It can be easy to carry over responses to one person and bring them into the next counselling session with another client. It is hard to avoid this with 15-minute gaps sometimes; even harder in some settings where it is like a conveyor belt with no time to quite literally 'collect yourself'. This is particularly so in medical settings where there is often little time between patients. Think of the GP surgery, patients coming in one after another. And even where there is a time gap, some other well-meaning member of the primary care team may grab the opportunity to ask the GP a question. I know, I have done it myself, waiting at the GP's door for a patient to come out so I can duck in and ask my question!

Another important aspect of a collaborative review process is that it offers the opportunity for the practitioner to talk through difficulties with clients ('I feel as though I have to have all the answers, but I know I don't, the fact is he is unlikely to get better'); or stresses that arise from clients who present with distressing symptoms ('sitting with her in that pain and feeling so utterly helpless, I just carry it for days'); or whose level of neediness drains the practitioner and reduces their effectiveness in establishing a therapeutic relationship with clients ('I just feel like a chewed rag after being with him, I think I'm losing my boundaries somewhere').

I would suggest, as well, that this form of supervision also has application in management. Again, managers are affected by their staff and may need reflective space to explore and understand the processes that shape their reactions. It can offer the possibility of greater self-awareness and more effective relationships with staff. Managers are required to treat staff fairly and equally, and the effective manager seeks to enhance the potential of their staff. A collaborative review process incorporating person-centred principles and practice will enhance a manager's ability, as a person, to work with their staff to meet the demands of the organisation and ensure that cultures of discrimination and bullying are given no opportunity to assert themselves.

It is my belief that a form of collaborative review along the lines I have highlighted should be accepted and established for all who work in therapeutic/healing/medical/nursing relationships. From the junior doctor on the busy intensive-care ward to the nurse visitor providing care for the elderly; from the aromatherapist working from home to the reflexologist working at a complementary health centre; and from the counsellor in any setting to the psychiatrist and community psychiatric nurse supporting the mentally unwell in the community – we all need person-to-person support and an opportunity to collaboratively review our work with clients. I believe that it serves to inform practice and enhance the practitioner's potential in their work. A psychologically healthy practitioner is going to be more effective in helping their clients. The qualities, attitudes and values of the person-centred approach as a model for supervision offer a powerful methodology for ensuring quality and effectiveness of practice, and greater wellbeing and personal development in the practitioner. This has to be for everyone's benefit.

Themes in the book

Supervision can encompass a range of themes and in this book I seek to demonstrate how particular issues related to the client's presenting problem(s) and their impact on the counsellor, can be usefully addressed in supervision. Chapter 1, through the process of supervising the counselling of a young person at a youth counselling agency, the therapeutic conditions are reflected on along with dealing with material that gets in the way, for instance, the impact of the supervisee's own childhood experiences. Chapter 2 offers a supervision session where the counsellor is working with a young person in a school setting. The primary issue is bullying and the supervision takes the supervisee back to his own experience of witnessing bullying as a child, and causes the supervisor to connect to her own experience of being victimised.

The supervision session in Chapter 3 deals with supervising a counsellor working with a person with an alcohol problem. It reflects on a session which the client's wife attended. Issues dealt with include the tendency to take sides. In Chapter 4 the supervision of a supervisee who is counselling a sexually abused client is presented. The supervision session includes processing the client having connected to herself as a little girl, and realising that the supervisee had missed something in the session. It also includes planning for when the counsellor is away on holiday, and in this instance the supervisor provides a point of contact for the client. A telephone conversation between supervisor and client is included in the chapter.

Chapter 5 deals with supervising the counselling of a client facing the diagnosis of a progressive disability. The counsellor explores her reactions and feelings to his struggle and relates back to an early life experience of her own. This leads on to Chapter 6 in which the focus is on supervising a counsellor whose client is coming to terms with having to accept her need to use a wheelchair. The counsellor uses supervision to explore his feelings towards his client and an experience in a counselling session in which the client experiences 'body-mourning' for the losses it has had to endure. In both these supervision sessions, issues of working with clients in physical pain are also addressed. This is not an easy issue to deal with and one that can arouse challenging reactions amongst supervisees.

We move to a GP surgery for Chapter 7 where the focus is on supervising time-limited counselling for stress. The impact of time-limited work is explored as it affects a client's decision to return to work, and a sense of weightiness in the counsellor's body is also explored to find its relevance for the counselling relationship. Chapter 8 provides a supervision session from a process of counselling a young man who is seeking to find identity and independence. In this session a particularly difficult and traumatising childhood experience is processed and the supervisee's feelings towards his client become a focus.

Chapters 9 and 10 are taken from a dual process. Chapter 9 is supervising the counselling of a muslim mother who is struggling to cope with her son's cannabis use and mental health symptoms, involving exploring issues connected with ethnicity and diversity and the application of person-centred theory. Chapter 10 provides an exploration of working in areas that may be at the limit of, or beyond, the supervisee's experience, supervising a late teenager experiencing psychotic symptoms associated with cannabis use. In some ways both these chapters are quite heavy, but the issues being addressed are serious ones, multi-faceted, and in many ways quite challenging. Working with people who struggle to cope with what has become termed as a 'dual diagnosis', will have a profound impact on the counsellor, and this in turn will influence the 'tone' of the supervision sessions. In particular, working with clients at the psychotic edge can be confusing, disorientating and difficult to follow in terms of the flow.

Chapter 11 explores issues arising in the context of supervising the counselling of a recovering drug user, and includes parallel processing, use of empathy, 'configurations' and 'parts', role reversal in supervision, and the need for recreational activities to augment supervision in order to restore wellbeing in the supervisee.

I end with my reflection on the writing of this book, and a short piece based on Rogers' 'Qualities of the person of tomorrow'.

CHAPTER I

Supervising the counselling of a young person at a youth counselling agency*

The dialogue introduces the client, Jodie, who was originally brought by her mother after she had found indications that she was using cannabis. Sandy, her counsellor, has experience of substance misuse work and is discussing their first few sessions with Courtney, her supervisor. Like many young people, Jodie is having to cope with a range of issues including: parents, school, best friends, street cred and her developing drug use.

Supervision session

Supervisor: Courtney

Supervisee/Counsellor: Sandy

Client: Jodie

'I've got a new client at the Agency. 15 year old. Jodie. Referred by her mother really, she'd found cannabis in her bedroom. Anyway, Jodie didn't want to be there and made that pretty clear at the start, but the relationship has developed since then, although I'm not sure she'll come back after the last session.'
Courtney smiled. 'They don't often hang around, do they?'
'Well, it got uncomfortable for her and she's really caught between using cannabis with her friends, or not using/or cutting back and risking losing her reputation and stuff.'
'Yeah, important stuff. So how does it feel being in relationship with her?'

---

*Taken from *Counselling Young People: person-centred dialogues* (2004) by Richard Bryant-Jefferies. Radcliffe Medical Press, Oxford.

A key feature of person-centred supervision lies in exploring the relationship that the supervisee has with her client and the feelings, thoughts and experiences that the supervisee has within that relationship. The emphasis is on helping them to reflect on their congruence, the quality and nature of their empathy and their ability to be warmly accepting of the client, and what may interfere with any of these. The intention being to clarify and to ensure that the supervisee is able to offer those aspects of the 'necessary and sufficient conditions' for which she has responsibility.

'It feels good and it feels challenging. I nearly said "felt" which I guess reflects my uncertainty as to whether she will come back.'

Courtney was nodding, 'yes, that seems quite present'.

'I'm concerned and I guess I'm wondering how well I handled expressing that concern.'

'Can you say a little more?'

'Well, we got into exploring her cannabis use.' Sandy went on to describe the party and the effects the cannabis had had on Jodie the next day, and the dilemma she felt she was facing with her two best mates, Ally and Em over it. As she spoke, Sandy could feel a sense of heaviness in her, it just felt so weighty to talk about. She voiced this.

'OK, so as you talk about this dilemma you can feel a real weight. In you, on you, around you?'

'Inside me, here.' Sandy put her hand over her tummy, just below the solar plexus. 'Feels kind of bulky as well.'

'So, weighty, bulky, in this area.'

As Sandy focused on it she realised that it was changing, dissipating and becoming more of an all-over sensation, but more on the edges of her body. 'It's shifted. It's more a kind of weight, no, more a kind of pressure all over my skin but it doesn't feel like it touches my skin. Makes me feel quite lethargic.'

'Lethargic, sort of not feeling motivated?' Courtney wasn't sure about that as he said it, somehow it sounded like he was trying to hang his own meaning on what Sandy was trying to say.

'No, she's motivated, but ... I've switched to talking about Jodie, that's interesting. Wonder why I did that?'

'I wonder too.'

Sandy sat with her experiencing. She couldn't figure out why, but she had a clear image of Jodie sitting like she had for a lot of the sessions, sort of slumped in the chair, and picking at her nails. She described this to Courtney.

'That how you feel?'

'Yes, I guess it is, and I'm aware I feel quite tense as well, up here, in my shoulders.' She took a deep breath. 'Feels like I'm carrying something, something heavy.'

'Mhmm, I'm just wondering whether it was something you picked up when you were with Jodie.'

Sandy could still see Jodie sitting there, and the struggle she had had, saying how she couldn't change, that she shared everything with her mates. She thought about how the session had continued. How Jodie had switched into wanting to go, to get on and live her life. Shit, Sandy thought, she kind of left it behind, dumped the heaviness of it all on me, or at least I picked it up. Or did she just leave me more sensitive to my own stuff? 'You know, I don't know that I picked it up, but maybe she put me in touch with something in me. I don't know that I believe we pick up our client's stuff unless we have something that kind of resonates to it within ourselves. I'm wondering what it may be in me that kind of got triggered by her dilemma, the weightiness of her struggle to decide what to do.'

'OK, so the question is what might be present for you that in some way may be similar to, affected by, Jodie's experience in that session?'

Sandy felt an overwhelming urge to stretch, which she did, and it felt good. Her back had become really tight and it felt energising to just open her arms out and move her back muscles.

'That looked satisfying,' Courtney smiled.

'Yeah, felt like I needed to expand a bit.' She paused to think for a moment. She thought about herself at Jodie's age. 'I never got out and about like she does when I was her age. Seemed to be at home most of the time. We lived in a fairly remote area. Didn't get out to many parties, but had the occasional sleep over. Don't remember any drugs being around much though, just didn't really figure. Why did I stretch when you said about what might be similar in me to what Jodie was experiencing? She just seems so different, head strong, out and about. Me, I was quiet, never really defied anyone. She just seems such a contrast.'

Courtney nodded and was struck by the difference. He wanted to ensure that Sandy knew he had heard this. 'I'm really struck by the difference between you, a real contrast.'

'Yes.' Then a powerful thought struck her, and it was powerful. One of those thoughts that she kind of knew, but then suddenly she *really* knew, like it became very immediate, and very present.

Courtney noticed Sandy's expression change. She had suddenly frowned. 'Yes?', he asked.

'Part of me would have so liked to have been like her, but would have been scared to death at the idea as well.'

'She kind of reminds you of how part of you wanted to be, but that also scared you as well.'

Sandy nodded. She could see some of the girls from her school, they just seemed so care free, so liberated, she couldn't think of a better word, just seemed to have a 'not care' attitude to life. She had always been so serious, and a little bit timid.

'I'm just thinking about some of the other girls at school and how they just seemed so cool, so . . . the word I had was "liberated", kind of freed up and confident. I was never like that, not really until I got into counselling. The training and the therapy changed all that.'

'But there is something about Jodie that kind of echoes from your past, of looking up to the other girls and wishing you were like them.'

'You know, I'm beginning to wonder if being with Jodie has kind of burst a bubble for me.'

Courtney frowned, unsure what Sandy was meaning.

'It's like maybe I've been carrying a secret desire to be like those girls, like Jodie is, at least, part of me has been carrying that dream, hope, call it what you will. And now Jodie has kind of burst it, shattered the dream. Made me, well that part of me, realise that maybe it isn't so glamorous as I thought it was. Yes, the more I think about this, the more real it feels. Part of me I have carried, unnoticed, and it has taken Jodie to come into my life to draw my attention to it.'

'She's given you quite a gift.'

'Well, I've often thought about how two-way this counselling is, how both the counsellor and the client learns through the process.'

> It does seem that counselling is a two-way process, that whilst the counsellor is offering an opportunity to their client, the client is generally offering something back to the counsellor as well. It can be helpful in supervision to reflect on what 'gift' the client has given the supervisor in terms of their experience of being with that client.

'Mhmm. So Jodie represents a dream that you have carried, kind of unwittingly, and suddenly the dream is seen through, no longer so glamorous.'

'No. And it seems to have left me more acutely aware of the risks that Jodie is taking, and I kind of feel that really did affect the way I was with her. I think I was maybe more concerned than I was aware of. I mean, she's not going psychotic on the cannabis, she's not smoking that much but she didn't feel good after that spliff she smoked and maybe if she carries on, and maybe they smoke more, well, I guess I'm concerned. I know I'm concerned. Shit there's part of me that wants to say, "for fuck's sake, Jodie, stop before it gets to you".'

'But you didn't say it?'

'No, and I don't know how much of that I was consciously aware of at the time, but I can certainly feel it now, and I'm left wondering if I'll see her again and whether an opportunity to make a difference in her life has been lost. And I really feel that.'

'Heavy feeling, huh?'

'Shit yeah, that's what it is. Yeah.' In that moment it felt like something had shifted and lightened inside herself. There was something about being able to acknowledge it, but she was also aware of feeling angry with herself as well, and aware that she wanted to trust Jodie, to trust her own process. But the truth was, she knew she didn't, at least she didn't trust it to keep Jodie safe. And that was what she was feeling more than anything else. Whilst she didn't have children herself, she felt that she wouldn't be letting her do what she did without saying anything. Oh-oh. 'I think I have the capacity to be too much like Jodie's mother.'

'You look shocked.' Courtney responded to Sandy's facial expression.

'Well, I began wanting to form a relationship with Jodie. I didn't know anything and just felt that here was another young person who wasn't understood and was being taken to us to be "sorted out" and "told what to do". Which we don't do. But now, I think I have a lot more sympathy for the mother. Well, I mean, I seem to have feelings for both Jodie and her mother now, and I can just see the fix they are in. Her mum must be exasperated, and Jodie is just, well, potentially heading for problems if she is particularly sensitive to cannabis, or it leads to other, harder drugs. Not that it started with the cannabis, she's already smoking tobacco and drinks alcohol, so she was already on the conveyor belt of mood-altering substances.'

'There seems to be a kind of inevitability in your voice, and I'm unclear where that's coming from. Not everyone does develop huge hard-drug problems from this kind of origin, though we know that many do.'

Sandy thought about it. She remembered something. 'Drugs are too close, too available. They get the cannabis from the brother of one of her friends, Ally I think, but I'm not sure. And that sense that they do everything together. I feel concerned that Jodie might have more problems with the substances. And I may be wrong, but it's what I sense, what I feel.'

'And it's important to acknowledge that, and I want to say that I really feel for you sitting with all these feelings, and I want to ask what you want from me to be able to, I don't know, manage, process – what's the right word? – *be* with what is present for you.'

Encouraging the supervisee to reflect on their supervisory needs is important. The person-centred supervisor will want to be open to what their supervisee feels they need, and seek to offer this where possible.

'I think having the space to just be with all of this, but in awareness, not having it on the edge and sort of unknown to me, is hugely important. I feel I'm kind of owning myself, my reactions, and that feels important. Like I don't want to go back to being with Jodie with a load of stuff on the edge of my awareness that impacts on our relationship and I'm not conscious of the process. I want to be congruent, authentic. I want to know myself accurately when I am in the room with her, you know? I don't want stuff going off inside me that disrupts my congruence or distorts my ability to accurately hear what she is saying and communicate what I have heard. I want to ensure that I can be warmly accepting of her and not let some reaction in me to her behaviour get in the way of that. Yeah, I don't mind not feeling good about what someone is doing, but I still hope to feel warm towards them, as the unique person that they are.'

Sandy could feel herself becoming more passionate as she was speaking. She cared, she really did care about her clients. She wanted to be authentically present for them, and for herself. She knew she felt more satisfied in her own experience of herself when she felt she was being authentic. She believed in those necessary and sufficient conditions, she knew from experience that they challenged the client, and the therapist, in so many ways, providing a relational climate within which constructive personality change could occur.

Courtney felt wonderful listening to Sandy connect with her passion and her belief in the approach. She just seemed to come alive, such a contrast again to how she had been a few minutes before, struggling with the heaviness of it all. He wanted to support her in this, acknowledge her strength of feeling. He knew he could say something jokey, but he also knew that would take away from the seriousness of the moment. Sandy was serious about her commitment to this way of working and he wanted to acknowledge the strength of that, support it, nourish it, encourage it. 'I'm really touched hearing you speak like that, puts me in touch with my own passion, but I want to honour yours. I want to say that Jodie has been lucky to meet you and I'm sure that you have affected her, even though she may not be aware of it. She's struggling with some really huge issues, particularly her street cred and being part of things with her mates. Hugely important stuff. You've listened to her, genuinely, and you've cared about her. Part of her may react against it, but other parts will recognise it like the seedling recognises which direction the sun is in.'

Sandy felt her eyes watering, particularly as she could see water in Courtney's eyes too. She swallowed. 'Thanks for that. Thanks. That image of the seedling, yes.' She blew out a deep breath, and she remembered something else from the sessions. 'I told her that I cared, I think it was in the second session. I forget how it came about, but it had a dramatic effect. It was one of those electric moments, and Jodie cried. She really heard and felt that care, I think. It really affected her. She said no one had ever expressed caring for her quite like that. It seemed to calm her, and she even said she felt more understanding towards her mother, acknowledged how much of a pain she must be to her mother.'

'Powerful, powerful stuff. You really connected with her.'

'Yes, but now she's disconnected.'

'From?'

'Me.'

Courtney could sense Sandy blaming herself, though she hadn't said it, it was the way she bit her lip after her response. 'Who's problem is that? Maybe she needs to ... for now. Part of her may feel threatened by the powerful experience she had with you. But she has felt your care, part of her has felt that, and that part won't forget it.'

Sandy nodded. 'Sown a seed, I guess.'

'And it will want to look for the sun.'

Sandy smiled, 'yeah, but there are some chemicals around that may destroy that seed, Courtney, it may not get a chance to germinate, that's what worries me.'

Courtney nodded, 'yeah, and there is no answer to that one. That's the tough realisation we all have to face, particularly working with people starting out using substances. How will they grow and develop, how much can they realise their potential as people, and what part will the substances play in that, either negative or positive?'

'Yeah, I know, so much creativity in our world has been drug induced – how many classical composers used substances to heighten their experience to pour into their music, and not just classical, of course?'

'And poetry, and art, and all kinds of creativity.'

'But I also see the damage as well, the fall out, the wasted opportunities, and with new substances being designed, we don't have a clue what the long-term effects are.'

'And so many young people don't live in a long-time time-frame. Those that do may have greatest resilience, but those who are into the experience of the moment, and that may be because what they see ahead is bleak and unacceptable, or it may simply be they want to feel good now and have found a fast way to achieve it chemically, they're not in touch with the idea of potential or actual long-term effects.'

Sandy nodded. 'I can feel quite depressed by it all at times.'

'You work in a tough environment, emotionally demanding. You care and you are effective because you care, but you are also affected because you care. But that care reached out and touched Jodie, and she won't forget that. It's gone in deep.'

'I need to hang on to that. Thanks for reminding me. I just wish I knew what was going to happen next, but then, maybe I don't. I just hope she turns up for the next appointment.'

'Yeah, you really do want that, I hope so too, and if she doesn't, well, maybe she has a good reason and she will get back in touch for more of that sunlight.'

Points for discussion

- How would you sum up the content of the supervision session? Were the issues covered that in your view needed to be?
- Evaluate Courtney's responses to Sandy. Was he staying with a person-centred philosophy of working?
- After reading through the supervision session, are you left feeling differently about Jodie, Sandy, young people, drug use? And if so, what is that difference?
- Reflect on the importance of the supportive element as a feature of supervision.
- Write your own notes for this session as if you were the supervisor.

CHAPTER 2

Supervising the counselling of a young person in a school setting*

Simon is the counsellor and he is working with Nick, a young teenager who is struggling with problems of bullying at school. Simon's supervisor is Sarida. Simon is an experienced school counsellor with a particular talent for engaging and working with young people. He sees clients during the day. Simon had recently given a talk about counselling at a school assembly and it had left Nick feeling that he could talk with him. However, at his first appointment Nick had not attended, shying away at the last minute. The young people have to get permission to take time out from lessons.

Supervision session

Supervisor: Sarida

Supervisee/Counsellor: Simon

Client: Nick

'I want to spend the last 20 minutes talking about a new client, a young lad at the school who I saw for the first time last Thursday.' Simon always wanted to at least check in with new clients as soon as possible in supervision, to first of all keep his supervisor up to date on who he was seeing, but also to use it as an opportunity to pick up anything related to how he was reacting to the client and the impact it could be having on the quality of the therapy he was offering. Often he didn't feel he had anything specific to raise, but that wasn't the case with Nick.

'OK, so, what do you want to tell me?' Sarida left it open for Simon to speak as he felt he wanted to. She trusted him to know if he had something he needed to

---

*Taken from *Counselling Young People: person-centred dialogues* (2004) by Richard Bryant-Jefferies. Radcliffe Medical Press, Oxford.

say. He seemed to come across to her as so sensitive to the kids he worked with, not just as a counsellor, he also occasionally spoke about his own children. He just seemed so cut out for working with them somehow, had that touch that you can't learn in books, and probably not learn on training courses either. It seemed to her that with some people what they needed most from counselling training was an opportunity to enhance their self-awareness, do work on themselves so that they could be authentic and congruently aware. She momentarily thought back to her own training and all the encounter groups that had helped her so much in coming to know herself. It had been tough, being Asian and Muslim. She had been the only non-white on the course, but she'd stuck it out and it had really helped.

People like Simon were natural listeners and seemed able to relate to people as easily as breathing. He seemed to have boundless warmth for the kids he worked with as well. And she knew that if he had something to say, if something hadn't felt right in the sessions, he would be keen to get a handle on it.

Simon began by describing Nick and then moved on to the issue and its impact on him. 'It's bullying, verbal, he's getting a lot of it, poor kid, and he doesn't know what to do.' Simon shook his head. 'But what he is doing, is using computer games to kind of release his pent-up feelings, at least, that's how it's coming across. You know, those games where you're killing people all over the place – bloody scary things for kids to get addicted to, but anyway, that's another rant for later. He's using them and imagining he's blasting the bullies. In a way, it kind of feels like a healthy psychological process in that it is at least helping him to release, but it's also getting him into a particularly murderous frame of mind.'

Sarida was aware of how fast Simon was talking. 'Really fires you up, yes?'

Empathic responses are not always directed by the content of what is said, the tone of what is said is also a key aspect of what is communicated. The supervisor identifies this, offering an opportunity to explore it further.

'Too right, and I know it's getting to me. I've seen a few kids this term with different kinds of bullying problems, but this one has got to me, and I know it's partly the computer games thing. Nick seems a bit of a loner, you know. Most of the others I've seen seem to have close friends and family they've talked to. But Nick doesn't.'

'So the other kids have talked to their parents but not Nick, and the computer games are leaving you feeling ... ?' Sarida left the sentence open, not sure quite how it was leaving Simon feeling.

'I feel for him, and I feel for the fact of what he is having to do to cope, which I don't think is healthy, but I guess it's helping him or he wouldn't be doing it, you know?' Simon was aware of feeling unsettled in himself, and he voiced this. 'It leaves me feeling unsettled.'

'Unsettled?' Sarida was wondering what Simon was meaning and in the back of her mind was what impact it would be having on the quality of his empathy for Nick.

A very brief response yet one that captures the primary feeling that is present for the supervisee, again offering the opportunity for the supervisee to connect more fully with what is present for them and to explore their experience.

'Yeah, kind of uneasy. That sort of churning kind of sense in my stomach. I mean, part of me feels that at least Nick is coming and he seems to be engaging. Oh yes and he was suddenly visibly brighter when we arranged for future sessions to be during his lunchbreak – giving him a break from the verbal bullying. Yes, I'd forgotten that. He really changed, he was suddenly so different and whilst I kind of acknowledged it, it was right at the end of the session. He must have been so aware of how it felt and I just wonder how long that lasted, and how he was then left feeling once the verbal started again, you know? I mean, he could feel a little more resilient, but he might find the contrast really difficult to handle.'

Sarida nodded. She was quite calm by nature and she was very conscious of how Simon was presenting. She wouldn't go so far as to say agitated, but he was animated. She wasn't feeling that way at all. She felt for Nick. She knew what bullying could be like as well. She had had a tough time at school as a Muslim. All kinds of names. She'd not been hit, but she'd been spat at and she had spoken about it at home but had not got any sympathy. Rather it was explained to her that it was something to be proud of, and that she should take the abuse for the glory of her religion. Looking back now she didn't agree. It was abuse and steps should have been taken. But that was then. She was very different now. She had moved on though she knew that she still carried sensitivities from those times.

'I was just being aware of my own experience, but also wanted to acknowledge my sense of your animation. There is something about Nick that has really touched you, Simon, and I am wondering what impact that is having on your empathy, your congruence, and whether your positive regard might be at risk of being conditional in some way.'

'I'm also aware that I drifted away from him a few times as well, caught in my own thoughts. On one occasion thinking back to my own childhood experience, about someone I remembered who was bullied at the school I went to.' Simon paused for a moment, consciously bringing his thoughts back to Nick. 'It's a real theme at the school where I'm counselling Nick. I did mention to him, no, he suggested it although I was thinking about it, about maybe mentioning it to someone. He was at first momentarily quite enthusiastic, but then he lapsed back into silence and said he was concerned what would happen if the ones who were bullying him found out that he had talked about it. So I said I wouldn't say anything at this stage. He seemed OK with that.'

'So he seemed OK with you not mentioning it. And what about you?'

'Me?'

'Mhmm. How do you feel having agreed not to mention it to anyone at the school?'

Supervision can develop as being very much centred on the client, however, the person-centred supervisor is also concerned about the impact of the therapeutic relationship on the supervisee, and on the therapeutic relationship they are creating with their client. The supervisee is enabled to understand themselves and their reactions more clearly, uncovering areas of unrecognised incongruence that might impact on the quality of their empathy. The result is a counsellor who can be more fully and clearly present with their client, able to respond accurately to what is being said with the minimum of interference from material within their own experience that is irrelevant to the client's inner world.

Shit, thought Simon, I hadn't really thought about that. He was suddenly aware that that uneasy feeling had returned and his arms felt a funny kind of tingling sensation. 'Uneasy. That feeling again.' He stopped and thought about it. What was he feeling? Where was he feeling it?

'Mhmm. That uneasy feeling again. Makes you feel uneasy knowing you've agreed not to say anything.'

He nodded slowly, looking into Sarida's eyes as he did so. He swallowed. 'It feels a heavy uneasiness, like it's heavy in my stomach.'

'Heavy like you feel full?'

'No. Just heavy, but moving, churning, like something soft and heavy just churning around inside me.'

'Soft and heavy, churning around inside you.' Sarida kept her response simple and focused to allow Simon to connect more deeply with what he had just conveyed to her.

Simon took a deep breath and let the air out slowly. Ian came back into his mind again, the kid from his school that was bullied. He could see him clearly, standing there on the school playing fields, being laughed at and jeered by the other kids. He was with them, but he wasn't joining in. God it was clear in his mind. He hadn't thought about that incident in years. He could remember walking away, walking away, having to get away.

Sarida sat with the silence that had arisen, maintaining her focus on Simon and awaiting whatever he felt he wanted to say. She commented, 'you look suddenly a long way away', which was how he felt to her, somehow strangely distant.

Sarida is responding to her experience of Simon as he sits looking distant, again, not a focus on what is being said but more on his way of being.

Simon nodded. He had heard Sarida but he didn't feel any great motivation to respond. He was somehow held by that past experience. It wasn't that he was remembering anything else, rather he had stopped remembering anything, he just felt stuck, somehow, powerless to move on. He was suddenly aware that his eyes were watering and he looked up, taking another deep breath.

'I was reliving an incident at school. The lad, Ian, was verbally taunted. I can see it happening and I remember walking away. I hadn't joined in, but I was with those who were doing the jeering. But I left. I just couldn't stay.' He tightened his lips. 'As I'm speaking now I've just flashed back to one moment, before I walked away. He caught my eye. I walked away, Sarida, I walked away. I couldn't do anything. I felt utterly powerless.' He shook his head. 'I couldn't ... oh shit ...'

'You couldn't ... ?' Sarida responded, speaking softly, not wanting to disturb Simon from what he was re-living. He was clearly connecting with some powerful feelings that he hadn't perhaps engaged with for a while. Certainly he had not talked this way before in relation to other clients at the school.

Simon shook his head and smiled, although it was a weak smile. 'I was about to say that "I couldn't stomach it". Yeah, I couldn't and at some level I still can't. The not being able to do anything. It's a big part of my motivation in what I do. And I know it but somehow it has become very real for me today.'

'Nick's helplessness has touched into your helplessness?' Sarida regarded her response as one of informed speculation.

Sarida has got a little ahead of Simon here, making a connection for him that perhaps would have been more valuable for him had he made the connection from the focus of his experience of helplessness. However, Simon can acknowledge this and continues to explore his experience.

Simon nodded. 'Yeah. That's what's got to me. And I know it's about the question of "will counselling be enough?". Should I do more? And part of me wants to do more. Part of me! It's a damn big part of me wanting to do more. Yet I also want to help Nick find his own voice, his own strength as well. I really want for that to happen.'

'Really want Nick to find his own voice, his own strength. That's a real goal for you, yes?'

Simon agreed. 'Yes, my goal, my goal. Shit. What a mess. I mean, there's me wanting to do more, wanting to do something to make a difference, a real practical difference with crap he's having to put up with. And there's this other part that has goals for him. I'm person-centred. I don't have goals.'

'Really?' Sarida knew she was playing devil's advocate. She knew that counsellors have goals, whatever their theoretical base. Even achieving psychological contact with a client is a goal.

'Yeah, I know. I think he's hooked that helplessness. I'm left realising how much that may be part of my motivation in this work. I mean, I kind of knew it but it's like I sort of know it even more now, and need to watch it because it will affect, does affect, no, has affected how I am. I can't push. I have to accept Nick where he is, and I have to carry that tension in me of wanting to alert the school but also wanting to maintain a confidential space for Nick. He made it clear he didn't want me to say anything and I feel I must respect that. He may change his mind and I hope he does, and I've got to be sure I don't encourage this. I really have to watch that.' Simon glanced at the clock. 'Time's getting on. And I haven't had a chance for my rant at computer games. Oh well, another time maybe.'

'I want to acknowledge that it seems that rant would be important for you, but I also want to check out where you are now given what we have talked about.'

'I need to really be there for and with Nick. I'm sensitive to the helplessness, of my own past powerlessness and I mustn't try compensating for that in my work with Nick. He has to travel at his pace. I have to give him my attention and offer him a supportive relationship and help him, well, help him whatever he needs to do to come through this with some degree of psychological health. And as I say that the thought of him spending hours on a computer fantasising about blasting the bullies to kingdom come doesn't feel healthy at all. But I have to hold that, it's my stuff. He's doing what he needs to do at this time and maybe if I can give him quality time and attention he may need less of that and begin to explore other ways of coping or dealing with the situation. I hope so. But I must accept him and not try and change him to fit my prejudices.'

The supervision session drew to an end. Simon felt much clearer in himself as he left although he was also aware of the effects of the intensity of the session. He felt sharper and drained at the same time. He took it steadily as he drove home, aware that he was lost in thought and having to make the effort to concentrate. Yes, he thought, Nick needs some space, his space, and he doesn't need it full of my attitudes and compensations for my past experiences. He felt determined to offer Nick a quality, therapeutic relationship and allow him to decide his focus and the pace. Yeah, he somehow felt he had reconnected with the attitudinal values and principles of person-centred working, and that felt good. He felt more positive. The uneasy feeling had passed. Yes, he thought, I'm going to help Nick find his way through all this.

Points for discussion

- How would you describe the tone and nature of the supervisory relationship between Sarida and Simon?

- Contrast this session with supervision as you have experienced it.
- What were the key factors in this supervision session?
- How did Sarida demonstrate her person-centred way of working in this session?
- If you had to choose a word or words other than 'supervision' to describe this process, what would you use?
- Write supervision notes for this session.

CHAPTER 3

Supervision of a counsellor working with a person with an alcohol problem*

Not every counsellor feels competent or confident towards the task of working with a problem drinker, and not all supervisors feel they have the knowledge to adequately support a supervisee working with this particular client group. There seems to be a kind of myth that drinkers are different – well, drinkers who have crossed that invisible line that defines whether their drinking is to be defined as problematic, often attracting the label of 'alcoholic'.

Not all problem drinkers are alcoholics. The degree that the drinking is a problem varies. It is not always about the quantity consumed. This can be the case in relation to health, and whether someone is free of alcohol in their bloodstream in order to drive or to work, but it is often more about the behaviours that result from the drinking, or the social, economic or legal costs that can follow. For instance, a person may only drink a couple of cans of lager. Is that a problem?

Well, if they then go on duty in a place of work where there is a no-alcohol policy, then yes, it is a problem. Or if the cans are strong lager (9% lagers in 500 millilitre cans are 4.5 units per can which is likely to be close to or over the legal drink-driving limit and above daily recommended safe drinking).

What does the supervisor need to know in order to be able to work with a counsellor who is seeing a client with an alcohol problem? I think some basic knowledge and understanding of how alcohol can affect a person, and the kind of behaviours that can arise, is important. Also the kind of concerns that might be present in the counsellor, and how these might impact on their work with the client. Some counsellors may feel unsafe, or may feel unsure whether counselling is actually helpful whilst a person is still drinking heavily and at times coming to sessions to some degree alcohol affected.

It is my experience that clients can be worked with, even when alcohol affected, and I have been amazed at times as to how much is recalled at a following session. This is not always the case; alcohol does affect memory, and people do experience

---

*Taken from *Problem Drinking: a person-centred dialogue* (2003) by Richard Bryant-Jefferies. Radcliffe Medical Press, Oxford.

alcohol blackout, which means they remain conscious and active during a period of time but the memory of what they are doing is somehow lost, or stored in the brain in such a way that it cannot be accessed later, hence the sense of having lived a period of time but with no awareness of exactly what happened.

For the person-centred supervisor, a key area to focus on with the counsellor will be congruence. Alcohol affects congruence. It disrupts the central nervous system and the processing of experiences. Congruence is a free flow of awareness between experience, awareness and communication (Bryant-Jefferies, 2001). Alcohol can affect a person's ability to be aware of experiences, and/or communicate accurately what they have experienced or what they are aware of. It is a suppressant, it depresses mood, affecting how a person may react to events. It can dampen down emotions, though it can also put people in touch with aspects of themselves as well, typically the person with suppressed anger whose alcohol use triggers a state of mind and emotion such that they are more prone to violent outbursts. The link between heavy alcohol use and violence is clear, and not just in terms of city-centre binge drinking. Alcohol is a major, probably the major factor, in incidents of domestic violence.

So the person-centred supervisor, working with a supervisee who is counselling a client with an alcohol problem, will be seeking to ensure that congruence is being maintained and, where they suspect it may not be, drawing attention to it and offering the opportunity to explore what is occurring for the supervisee.

The following dialogue is taken from the third supervision session in relation to work being done with a particular client, Dave. The counselling takes place at an alcohol counselling agency. Dave began to attend counselling for his drinking at the suggestion of his GP. At the start, he did not think he had a problem, but he began to realise that it was causing him problems, and in particular in his relationship with his wife, Linda. Dave manages to cut down but it has not been easy, and his urge to drink is driven by earlier life experiences along with habitually going down to the pub.

In the previous supervision session, Alan, the counsellor, discussed with his supervisor, Jan, the possibility of Dave bringing his wife to a session. It was something that Dave had suggested after he had talked it through with Linda. She had planned to come to a previous session, but in the end had not made it. The idea was that it would be something of an information session – not unusual in alcohol counselling agencies. It would be an opportunity for Linda to understand firsthand what was being offered and for her to say anything she wanted to, as well as an opportunity to emphasise that a drinking problem within a relationship will need both people to work together to resolve it.

Dave has so far been offered seven sessions of counselling with Alan. He has attended six. The session he did not attend followed on from his having drunk heavily, been locked out and, as a result of a disturbance, spent the night in the police cells and had to sleep at a mate's house. Linda had made it clear that she did not want him back. Things had eased in the relationship since then, and they are now back together.

Alan attends the supervision session after having had a previous counselling session two days before at which both Dave and Linda were present. The session had been largely taken up with events that occurred at their son's birthday party which had happened a few days previously. Dave had been looking forward to this but the experience had triggered memories and feelings from his own childhood and had lead to him heading down the pub to be with his mates – and to have a few drinks.

Alan needs to update his supervisor, Jan, as to what is happening, and to talk through the session that Linda attended with Dave, and also some other experiences from two other sessions since the last supervision session. Two other areas that he needs to discuss are an experience of calmness that emerged for Dave during one of these sessions, and also an exploration of the sense of a deep, dark pit which Dave had described in the session but which Alan had not accurately responded to empathically. He wants to process this in order to be clear about what happened, why he responded the way that he did, and what he may need to address in himself in order to ensure he can accurately listen to and hear Dave in future counselling sessions.

Supervision session

Supervisor: Jan

Supervisee/Counsellor: Alan

Client: Dave

Client's wife: Linda

'Good job we talked about couple counselling last time', Alan said as he settled into the easy chair in the room that Jan used for her supervision practice. 'Not that it turned out how we discussed, and it did end up as couple counselling at times and not just information exchange, but it was very powerful and deeply moving. Made a big impression on me and left me feeling quite drained. I was glad to have given myself extra time after that session before the next person. I had half an hour and I really needed it.'

'So, what happened?', Jan enquired.

The supervisor has directed the counsellor towards describing events and has unwittingly avoided a focus on what the counsellor has said about feeling drained – the impact of the counselling session on him. Supervision should be ensuring that the counsellor is both supported and enabled to experience a certain degree of feeling restored. The supervisor could have embraced both areas that the counsellor has described, leaving him free to take his own direction, which would have been a more person-centred supervisory response. The counsellor, however, is strong enough to be able to defend this directive response as he is clear that he has things he wants to explore even though he is unsure where to begin. In fact he had already begun and if the empathy for what had been said had been offered, the counsellor might have flowed naturally into the themes he had already introduced. The supervisor later connects with the notion of not directing the supervisee, but it has already happened and has not been recognised. It would therefore be a supervisory issue for the supervisor, to explore and process why she chose at that moment to focus on the recalling of events rather than the effect that they had had on the supervisee.

'Dave came with his wife, Linda, but I am also aware that there were some other things that have happened in previous sessions that I want to talk about, so I'm not sure where to begin.'

Alan was thinking back to the sessions when Dave had experienced that dark pit and yet curiously how Dave had ended up with a strong sense of calm and of feeling OK. He wanted to check that assumption he had made about Dave being in the pit. And there was everything about the birthday party, Dave's confidence and his, Alan's, feeling that it was going to be a problem, as well as that session with Linda. The last session was fresh in his mind, but there was something about that calmness Dave had touched that was very present in his thoughts.

This may seem like a lot to take in, and it is. Counselling sessions can bring up a range of material for consideration and review in supervision, and it can be difficult to keep track of it and difficult for the supervisee to know just where to start.

Jan sensed that Alan was not sure where to start, she didn't want to direct him, but she wanted to acknowledge her sense. 'Seems like there is a lot of material and I guess it has made a strong impact on you. Hard to know where to start?', she asked, leaving Alan to pick up the story where he felt he needed to.

A much more clearly non-directive, yet empathic response. The supervisee can now proceed with what is most pressing for him, rather than feel pushed in a particular direction by the supervisor.

'So much seems to be going on for Dave at the moment, he really does seem to be moving across a whole range of experiences. It is almost as though he is connecting with parts of himself, and my sense is that there is some kind of process running here.'

'Some kind of process that is helping Dave feel more connected with himself?', Jan
asked wanting to be sure she was clear on what Alan was saying, and allowing
Alan to hear it himself so he could clarify anything that did not sound right.

'The session after the last supervision, Dave went into himself and into what he
described as being a deep, dark pit. I immediately thought he was descending
into some dark depth, and I remember responding: "A deep dark pit. You inside
it?" but he corrected me saying, "no, it's inside me". I had assumed it was his
whole self entering into a pit.'

'Any idea where that assumption came from? Can you remember whether you
felt connected with Dave at the time?' Jan was wondering whether Alan was
speaking from his own experience.

'I thought I was', Alan replied, trying to remember how he had felt.

Alan had spent time reflecting on this himself. He regularly used a period of
self-reflection to process his counselling work. He found this an important
discipline and aid to helping him understand his own process and what was
happening in the sessions rather than simply always waiting for the next
supervision session. He felt it was a responsibility of counsellors to self-monitor.
However, in this case he had struggled to get clarity as to his feelings and sense
of what had been happening in the session with Dave.

In many respects, an effective counsellor regardless of theoretical base must
develop within themselves a kind of internal supervisor. By this I do not
mean something that sits constantly in judgement – and if it took this form
then it would be a supervision and probably a therapy issue – but rather an
accepted element of their professional practice in which they would devote
time to reflect on the counselling process, and the effect that it was having on
themselves, and the client. Some people may use a process diary, others may
simply sit and reflect. Some counsellors may prefer to undertake this process
straight after a counselling session, others at the end of a day. There may be
a preference to do this in the counselling room, or to take the process into a
different space. The counsellor will choose their own style and method.
It should be noted that process diaries are part of a client's notes and would
be required to be submitted if a complaints procedure/litigation arose.

'What was being talked about before you made your assumption?'

'We were talking about how empty he would feel if he had to face not being with
his wife and children. It was emptiness that took him into the pit.'

'You are doing it again', Jan replied, 'talking of him going into the pit, even
though you say he said the pit was in him.'

'Dammit, something's going on here and I need to clear it.'

'Emptiness', Jan said it softly, 'where does emptiness take you?'.

Alan sat and thought, but not for long, he knew it was his own relationship break
up that had dropped him into the pit. 'It's my stuff. It was my experience, but
somehow at the time and after I didn't think of it, it just seemed so reasonable to

assume Dave as a whole was dropping into a pit', he said finally, feeling irritated that his own stuff was clouding his sensitivity to his client. Alan had not experienced this himself for some time, he had done a lot of work on himself in order to move on, yet it seemed some scars remained. 'It seems that even though I have come to terms with what happened, the intensity has left me with a kind of weak spot, and themes or feelings that come up, or become present and touch into this weak area, trigger this kind of assumption.' Alan was annoyed with himself.

It may seem that what is being explored is a small point, perhaps even a matter of language because at the end of the day the client is experiencing the presence of a deep, dark pit and the sense of this has been conveyed to the counsellor. But it didn't feel smooth for the counsellor, there felt a block to accurate hearing. A key element in effective counselling lies in ensuring that content within the counsellor's frame of reference does not intrude on the accurate hearing of what is present for the client. Clients can be despairing of anyone ever really hearing what it is like for them, and they don't need a counsellor who cannot hear what they are trying to convey because of their own issues and experiences. As is so often the case, in exploring the 'block' or mismatch in understanding, other themes emerge. Where something is not heard accurately there is often a good chance it is because something is present in the supervisee affecting the quality and accuracy of their listening, and the event has to be explored in order to connect with what lies behind it.

'You don't look very comfortable?', Jan replied, knowing that Alan set high standards for himself and that he didn't like to feel he was not clear in himself in his therapeutic work.

'I've been working on my sense of loneliness in therapy, and it has been really helpful. I am annoyed that something like this got past me. I'm going to look at this more, but not here. I am wondering, though, what reaction you have to this?'

'I'm sitting with a sense of just how close some of Dave's experiencing is to yours, and how you need to be aware of this in working with him. It seems as though Dave corrected you pretty quickly and no harm was done. He explained how it was and presumably you moved on into his world of experience. I am assuming, it seems assumptions are in the air today, that your assumption didn't stick with you.'

The theme of assumptions has now emerged. Counsellors have to be very sensitive to this, and their supervisors also. For the person-centred supervisor there will be an emphasis on ensuring that blocks to listening are dealt

> with. Often a person-centred supervisor will use their own experienced reactions to the supervisee as a way of recognising where something does not feel quite right. But they will need a high quality of congruence, of accurate self-awareness, to distinguish these elements. But where they are sensed then the supervisor has responsibility to voice them.

Jan noted how, in supervision, the supervisor could parallel in some way the issues within the counselling sessions. Her job was to try and notice these and highlight them. They often had meaning. Assumption seemed to be emerging as a theme and she wondered what relevance it may have both to Alan's relationship with Dave, and to Dave generally in his life. It sometimes felt like she was taking a position just behind the counsellor, ready to catch anything emanating from the client that the counsellor missed, yet holding a vantage point so that she might sense what impact the counsellor might be having on the client. Yet she knew, too, how reliant she was on the counsellor being open. Therefore she sought to create a collaborative environment so that she and Alan could work together as co-professionals, not in some kind of teacher–pupil relationship.

'It didn't stick. As I recall, Dave moved on and connected with the pit inside himself.'

'So how do you think the theme of assumptions may have relevance in your relationship with Dave, or in Dave's life in general?'

'I'm not sure. I was aware pretty quickly that I was making an assumption when it happened. I suppose when Dave spoke of his assumption that he would be OK at his son's birthday party.'

Jan looked curious, 'what happened with his son's birthday party?', she asked.

'Well this was the next session, his son was having a birthday party on the Saturday and Dave was looking forward to it, to giving his son the kind of birthday he didn't have as a child. I felt alarm bells and tried to voice my concern, but he would have none of it. He was sure he would be OK. He assumed he was going to be able to cope.'

'And did he?', Jan knew the answer before she asked the question.

'Well, he used alcohol to cope, let's put it that way, and the last session with Linda was following the birthday party. Dave had been affected and had felt an urge to be with his friends seeing his son having fun with his friends and in particular when sides were being picked for a team game, it took him back to his own painful memories of not being picked 'till last. Dave ended up in the pub, drinking heavily, and it triggered a relapse for a few days back to pub drinking. Before then he had got it back under some degree of control and was working at cutting back further.'

'So, Dave made an assumption about his ability to control his drinking in what must have been a difficult situation at some level for him. Maybe he makes assumptions about a lot of things? It may be something to be aware of and which may need to be highlighted if it feels to be a factor when you are with him again.'

Jan didn't want to suggest Alan raises it as, like Alan, she did not believe in being directive and going into sessions with a pre-planned list of items to raise. So often clients have moved to a different place and the person-centred approach honours this. She believed things should be raised when they were felt to be part of the therapeutic process. She strongly liked the concept of transparency as a description of congruence and the ability of the therapist to voice experiences that became present within them during, and as a product of, the therapeutic relationship.

Person-centred counselling is a dynamic, relational process. The factor of immediacy in the sense of attending to what becomes present when it becomes present is highly significant. The person-centred supervisor will want to ensure that the supervisee, working from the same theoretical model, is staying with the client on their journey and being attentive to what emerges. Think of sharing a train journey with someone. One person looks out of the window and shares their impressions of the views as you pass together through the countryside. The other person listens, conveys what they hear they are being told and, at times, when something out of the window catches their eye in a way that it really stands out to them and stops them hearing the other person, may then comment on what they have seen. But not always. Sometimes it will need to be set aside.

If we think of this as a metaphor for supervision, it will be set aside to be explored later. Or it may be voiced if it really is 'in the way' and may be sensed as having therapeutic significance. Sometimes, in moments of deep connection with clients, the counsellor can experience urges to speak or act that may not seem explainable at the time, but turn out to be in some way right. So whilst the aim is to empathise, there will be times when transparency is called for, and the counsellor will need to make visible what has become present for them. But care must be taken, to ensure that what is voiced is limited to what has emerged into the person-centred counsellor's experience and does not extend itself into an interpretation of that experience.

'Yes, I think I need to carry a heightened awareness of it, and see what happens. The problem in this line of work, particularly with alcohol problems, is that people can easily make lots of assumptions. You only have to say the word "alcoholic" and a whole host of images can come to a person's mind that may have no relevance whatsoever to the person who is being referred to. And, of course, Dave's childhood was riddled with assumptions as he tried to make sense of his relationship with his mother. He clearly assumed that loneliness and rejection were somehow normal, or at least, normal for him to experience. The more I think about this now, the more this theme of assumptions makes sense. But not just for Dave. It is a factor for so many clients, well, for all of us, isn't it? We start making assumptions at such an early age as we try to make sense of our experiences.'

Alan was thinking of a number of his clients who had all made natural assumptions in childhood because of what they experienced of never being good enough or of not deserving to feel happy. This could be the result of many experiences, and themes that often emerge are: violence in the home, victimisation, physical and sexual abuse, lack of prizing or constant criticism.

> As children we receive a lot of negative experiencing that we try to make sense of, and often the sense that is made involves the belief that we deserve to feel hurt because of who we are, and this then becomes a 'configuration of self' within the individual's self-concept. This then fuels assumptions that we make about ourselves in later life, often resulting in a reinforcement of the original attempt to make sense of a dysfunctional situation.

It is always somebody else's 'good enough' that we are supposed to conform to, Alan thought, producing what Rogers termed conditions of worth. 'I'm thinking of conditions of worth', Alan added, 'and acknowledging their link with making assumptions.'

'How do you see or maybe I should say experience Dave's conditions of worth?', Jan asked.

'Nice one!', was Alan's instant response. So, what had Dave been conditioned into in order to feel some degree of worth? 'Well, he said he got no cuddles from his mother, no parties, no friends to speak of. He has also told me how he never got picked for teams at school, that he was always the last to be picked and really neither side wanted him. It must have seemed such an impossible idea for Dave to feel accepted, wanted, cared for. The more I think of it now, the more angry I feel about what he had to go through. I often think that if I had had the experiences of my clients maybe I would be drinking heavily to cope, and I certainly think that with Dave. With his background, I might have handled my relationship break-up last year in a very different way. Makes you think. Makes me feel quite humble, somehow.'

'Humble?'

'Maybe that's the wrong word, I don't know, but it makes me aware of just how fortunate I am and not because of anything that I kind of achieved. I didn't have Dave's early experiences and so I wasn't left with the sensitivities that he has, or at least not the associated habit reactions that he has with them of taking alcohol to quell uncomfortable feelings. Me, I just headed off to the gym and burned it off when I was struggling last year. But it could have been very different. Makes you think.' Alan sat for a moment, aware of how awesome this kind of thinking was.

'Makes *you* think', he heard Jan say. Yes it did make him think, it made him very aware that if life experiences had been reversed it could have been Dave counselling him for a drink problem!

Alan thought of a theme in the training workshops he ran on working with people with alcohol problems. 'One of the things I always try to get across in training is this idea that there is no *us and them* with problem drinking. We are all human beings trying to make the best of things, and some of us choose alcohol to help, because it eases the pain, or gives us a boost, or a good feeling.'

In supervising a counsellor working with people who have alcohol problems, it is important to avoid the 'they're different' trap. There is no 'us and them'. In reality we all make choices in order to try and feel different, usually to feel better which can mean feeling more connected with ourselves, or parts of ourselves, although it can also involve avoidance as well. People will define what better means based on their own life experiences which in turn shape their sense of what is normal for them, and what they seek to aspire to. Some people choose to drink to feel different, some climb mountains. Some people join a gym, still others read books or go to the cinema or theatre. We like to feel good, and for some that involves engaging with the familiar, maintaining habits. The problem with alcohol is that because it is an addictive substance, too much for too long leaves the person needing to take more in order to stave off withdrawal reactions which, in extreme cases, can be life-threatening. So there can be a desperate felt need to keep drinking to avoid this, which involves therefore feeling better in the short term even though longer term it is simply causing damage and increasing the risk of things becoming a lot worse.

Jan knew from past conversations that Alan felt this way, and she could sense his feeling for Dave. It was very present and she voiced it. 'You really feel for Dave, don't you?'

'I do, and it was very present for me when he was with Linda early on in the session. He had relapsed and she was giving him a hard time in the session. At the time I didn't appreciate her background and sensitivities. What I felt was that I wanted her to shut up and give Dave some space.'

'Sounds as though you were maybe being a bit protective of Dave against Linda?' Jan suggested.

That hadn't occurred to Alan. A broad grin broke out on his face, 'never thought of myself as a mother hen before', he replied and broke out laughing. 'But the session changed later and they really came together. It was very moving. Dave talked about his loneliness and the rejections he had had in childhood, particularly the experiences around not having friends, not being popular, and Linda talked of her father who had an alcohol problem and the arguments at home when he came back from the pub. They both heard things they hadn't heard before, and it really drew them together.'

'Sounds like a good piece of work.'

The supervisor has prized the supervisee, and this is important. But she has not registered Alan's wanting to be protective of Dave, and what message that may have communicated. He laughs off the notion of being a mother hen, but perhaps he is, perhaps he does know this but it is uncomfortable to engage with. Perhaps he feels he will be judged if he admits to it. We do not know, it has not been explored, but it arguably should have been. Alan may not have said anything in relation to feeling protective of Dave, but feeling it could have affected his facial expression or tone of voice. In a genuine couple counselling session the counsellor would not be taking sides, and if the urge to do so became present, they would need to explore this in supervision. The exploration in the counselling session when Dave and Linda talked about their pasts had been very moving and Alan had done a good piece of work with it. It really had helped to build a bridge between Dave and Linda.

'Didn't feel like work. I didn't really say much, or at least I don't remember it as though I did. I remember wanting to let them be in the moment, particularly when Dave reached out to take Linda's hand when she had been talking about how much fear she had linking back to her father going down the pub and coming back drunk, and how this connected to Dave going down the pub.' Alan sensed water in his own eyes as he related this part of the session. It had been so touching, and he felt as if he had somehow borne witness to something very precious taking place between Dave and Linda. 'Yeah, it felt good to be there with them, and at the same time part of me now wonders whether I should have left the room and let them just be together. Although I don't recall thinking it at the time, it could have become a bit voyeuristic somehow.'

'What was your anxiety, although I'm not sure anxiety is the right word?' Jan asked, sensing how moved Alan was and yet also a sense that he had maybe felt a little awkward. 'No, not anxiety, maybe awkwardness?'

'Not sure what I felt. It just seemed such a tender moment between them, it was a privilege to be there and I am just wondering . . . I'm not sure what I'm wondering, it's something about it all being very fragile and not wanting to kind of damage it I guess. I remembered a phrase from a little book at the end of the session: "Look for the flower to bloom in the silence that follows the storm: not 'till then". I had to look up the rest of the passage. There was something very beautiful about what happened between them. I hope it lasts but I fear that it won't.'

'Fear that it won't', Jan allowed herself to look puzzled. Alan had seemed so positive and yet now he was indicating he had doubts.

'Yes, I don't know, it's alcohol. When alcohol's in the picture you can just never be too sure what is going to happen next.' Alan knew only too well that the kind of experiences both Dave and Linda had been through had left them both vulnerable, and Dave's drinking could easily be triggered. He hoped it wouldn't happen, but he knew the possibility was there.

Jan had the word assumption in her head again and yet it didn't seem to fit. She knew too that where alcohol was concerned things were not always as they seemed, and that achievements were not always maintained. Yet she knew that people did change an alcohol habit, that they could move on. She sensed the stress in Alan as he stood between his conflicting feelings: the hope that what he had witnessed would last and flourish, and that it would help them both to resolve old patterns and drinking behaviours, and the fear that something would go wrong and that the part or parts of Dave's self-structure linked to his heavy drinking would fight back.

She remembered reading that article about the self-concept striking back, how when you change, the part of yourself that you are seeking to change or leave behind can seek to reassert itself (Mearns, 1992).

As we change, we develop new parts of ourselves (or modify existing ones), and fresh ways of being emerge as we see ourselves, our experiences and the world around us differently. The old parts can remain and fight back in order to restore their power and supremacy. This has particular significance when working in the field of addiction, whatever the addiction might be. The part, or parts, of the person that are associated with the addictive behaviour are strong. They have been established over time and will have become, for the person, their normal way of being. Experiences that take them into feelings associated with those parts can trigger the parts back into life, as it were, triggering a heightened risk of a relapse. For instance, someone who has been a pub drinker but has cut back or stopped and as part of this has avoided going into pubs, may find that the parts of themselves that developed in the context of pub life will re-emerge, and even after years, if that person goes into a pub. Memories surface in powerful ways as the person reconnects with aspects of themselves that they would have thought had been left behind. It is why people need to learn new behaviours, new responses to old and familiar alcohol-related settings and experiences. It is helpful for the supervisor to be mindful of this. The switch from a newly developed part into a previously established alcohol-associated part within a person can occur very rapidly.

'Alan, I'm just so aware of the tension between holding on to hope and acknowledging fear of further difficulties. You are concerned that Dave's drinking configuration (Bryant-Jefferies, 2001) is going to strike back, aren't you?'

'Yes. I don't think we have seen the last of Dave's "lonely me" configuration, and knowing the depth that it can take him to I am fearful.'

'Fearful of?' Jan asked.

'Not sure. If he was depressed I'd be concerned in case it might take him into a suicidal frame of mind. But he hasn't indicated this and I haven't felt any need to ask about suicidal ideation, it simply has not been presented from within his frame of reference, or a factor that has emerged within my own thoughts and feelings during our interactions. He was quiet in the session initially following his drinking last weekend and into this week, but he did not seem unduly depressed beyond what would be a natural reaction to what had happened. But I know the risk is there if someone really drinks heavily on desperate feelings. I just need to have it in mind, I guess, and I am also aware of a resistance in me to this because I don't want to start carrying that thought into the sessions. I certainly don't want to give him ideas.'

'You think that part of his self-structure, "lonely me", might take him into a suicidal frame of mind?'

'I don't know. I hope not, but I also have to be realistic. It sounds odd talking this way when the last time I saw them they seemed so close, and with so much hope between them to try and make things work and move on. And yet ...' Alan wasn't sure why he was feeling quite so apprehensive. Was it simply his knowledge and experience of working in this speciality that was triggering this, or was it something genuinely emerging as a product of the therapeutic relationship?

'And yet ...' Jan repeated, and a question instantly dropped into her mind. She voiced it. 'Do you routinely feel this way with clients in these kinds of situations?'

'No, and this is probably what is concerning me. I haven't anything to support my concerns, but they are very present. I think I need to see if this passes or whether it remains with me. If it remains a nagging concern then I want to say something at the next session, but I want it to be in the context of the interaction that we are having. I need to see whether this is still present next time and if so, if it is strongly present for me in the session, then I will say something. And I will trust myself to say it in a way that expresses my feelings at the time. I don't think a prepared intervention is helpful. I want to say what I need to say in a way that is kind of organic.' Alan felt he would be saying something, it did feel like it was going to persist.

'OK, I am sure you will find the right words in the moment, Alan. Trust your instincts.'

'Yes, this is the part of counselling that some people perceive as being a bit woolly, but we do end up time and time again trusting our instincts, trusting ourselves to be what is helpful within the counselling relationship. I know it is such a part of person-centred working, and I certainly can't pre-plan a session, I need it to flow out of the relationship I create with my client as I offer the core conditions. Dave had crap relationships as a child and he's been badly affected. My role is to offer him another experience and a chance to grow, to develop, to discover other ways of being as a result and to offer him the unconditional positive regard he didn't experience in early life.'

'Other ways of being which will become deeply satisfying to him as he recreates his self-structure in response to being in therapeutic relationship with you' Jan added.

'Yes, and in one sense it is simple although very difficult and painful in terms of the human experience, and there is the alcohol in the picture which we know can skew people's mood and leave them making destructive choices that they might not have otherwise made.'

'OK, so you will raise the issue of Dave's mood at the next session if your concerns persist?' Jan asked.

The supervisor has a responsibility both to the supervisee and to the client. The possibility of a suicidal frame of mind emerging within the client has become a possibility to the supervisee. He has nothing to base this on other than his own sense, and of putting experiences together that the client has described. It is good practice to ensure that a client feels safe with their mood and state of mind. A supervisor needs to support the supervisee in their chosen response to this kind of issue, allowing them time to explore what is happening, their options and their feelings. They may not be immediately aware of the full extent of the impact it is having on them, and time can be given to allow what is present to emerge more fully into the supervisee's awareness, enabling them to plan what their response might be.

The supervisee is encouraged to trust their own reactions, thoughts and inner experiencing – their 'internal locus of evaluation'. The person-centred supervisor will want to be sure that the supervisee has clarity within themselves as to what is occurring, so far as this is possible, and there will be times when there is no clarity, at best there is a 'felt sense' that something is occurring, or that there is potential for something to occur.

'Yes, and I rather feel that I will be raising it as I feel that my concerns are going to persist.' Alan could feel unease in his stomach as he said this. 'I can feel it in here', he said, patting his belly. 'I felt similar concerns at the end of the session before last concerning the birthday party, and I was right. I need to trust these feelings.'

Jan nodded, she trusted Alan. He was clearly concerned and she knew he would say something and in an appropriate and sensitive way. She was also aware that something was nagging at her. It was Alan's strong reaction to Linda when he experienced a wish that she would shut up and give Dave some space. She knew she needed to raise this.

'Alan, I'm stuck with something, with wondering what was happening for you when you said you were feeling that you wanted Linda to shut up and give Dave some space. It sounded intense and it feels as though there was a sharp edge to it somehow, or at least that is my wonder. It feels sharp and it is persisting in me.'

This is another key feature of person-centred supervision. The supervisor will trust their experience and, if they feel something has not been dealt with, or are left with a sense of something having been unresolved, they will want to make this visible. Here the supervisor trusts their 'internal locus of evaluation'. Something is not feeling right, has been left unresolved, and needs clarifying. Of course, if it turns out that whatever is raised by the supervisor is not significant then they will need to explore this themselves in their own supervision.

Alan thought for a moment. Yes, it had been a sharp moment. And once again Jan had picked something up on the basis that it was worrying at her. He liked her way of working, she trusted her experiences within the supervision relationship and usually when she voiced this kind of nagging discomfort it had value and importance.

'Mhmm, yes, that's what I like about you, you don't miss much! I had thought about this and I think I was feeling so close to Dave, so much striving to maintain connection with his inner world plus the history we already had, that I was feeling kind of protective.' Alan had felt Linda was crowding Dave and that Dave needed time to say what he needed to say. He felt he had been protecting Dave's right to say what he wanted to say, but he also acknowledged to himself that he had cut across Linda. 'It has also made me aware of how difficult it can be to work with a couple when you already have a therapeutic relationship with one of them. I want to take this into therapy and look at it more deeply as well. In thinking about it I had a sense that maybe I need to explore this in the context of whether it is a male/female issue.'

'Male/female?' Jan responded, hoping Alan would clarify this further.

'I just wonder if it was a male to male thing that was contributing to my need to maybe protect Dave, and/or whether Linda was hooking some strong feelings in me that were rooted in other experiences. I'm unclear about it at the moment, I just have this sense that I need space in therapy to go into it a little deeper and see what comes up. I want to check out whether my reaction is more than being simply a product of having a closer connection to Dave as a result of our work together over recent weeks.'

'What's your intuitive sense on this, Alan? I think you are right to use therapy to explore it, but I am wondering what you may be sensing within yourself about it.'

Jan wanted to encourage Alan to listen to his own inner prompting. She would always endeavour to be open to her own reactions and voice anything that she felt needed to be made visible, but she wanted Alan to put into his own words what he was sensing.

There sometimes needs to be an open discussion as to what needs to be dealt with in supervision, and what needs to be taken into therapy. Time can be a factor. If something deeply significant emerges for the supervisee that is affecting their counselling work, then it is likely that it must be taken to therapy, but with some agreement on reviewing progress in supervision.

In extreme situations it could be that a decision has to be reached as to whether a particular supervisee can continue to work with a client presenting with issues that are triggering their own unresolved material. Ideally, this should be a collaborative decision, however, there can be occasions when, in line with ethical frameworks and codes of practice, it is clear that work with a particular client has to stop or be suspended.

'I think it is simply my feelings towards Dave, but I am sufficiently uneasy about it to want to check this out. I think I was in touch with my sense of Dave's vulnerability and he was under pressure and not getting heard. I know I've felt unheard at times and I want to be sure it wasn't hooking this in some way. I want to be clear in myself and about myself. I want space to focus on me. Does that sound reasonable?'

Jan nodded her head. She wanted to encourage Alan to trust his own inner prompting so she responded, 'it seems you have thought this through and have a clear sense of what you want to do. I feel more at ease knowing you were aware of this issue and are taking steps to work on it, or at least clarify it for yourself. It obviously feels important to you to handle it this way'.

'Yes, it does. It seems right to take the emphasis on me to therapy whilst bringing here more of a focus on Dave and the relationship with him. I know it is hard to separate sometimes, it all seems a bit artificial at times and I often wonder whether the divide between supervision and personal therapy is actually helpful. Yet at the same time I acknowledge that without some kind of boundary the emphasis in supervision could become overly focused on the counsellor with little time for clients, and that wouldn't be helpful.'

'So, boundaries are important, and I agree. And your sense is that where the focus becomes too much on the counsellor then the boundary has slipped?' Jan asked wanting to check she was hearing Alan accurately.

'Yes, and I realise this is an area that in counselling and therapy we are more used to talking about whilst other professions may not recognise the need for personal work in the same way in order to work effectively with clients. A lot of people I know have line-management supervision which can offer little or no scope for any personal exploration. And clinical supervision which can be so focused on diagnosis and following procedures that the relationship gets lost somewhere. Yet for me, so many of the helping professions are about forming relationships with clients, and people are affected by this and do need to explore this. Well, that's what I think anyway. I've strayed back on to my soapbox again! But I do feel strongly that supervision is not well understood, and I think people need space to explore their personal reactions to client work and how they are affected by particular clients and the impact this has on their work with them. And when it becomes a personal issue for the professional involved then some kind of therapeutic work becomes necessary to ensure not only their mental and emotional health, but more importantly that of the client.'

The supervisee is raising an important point. How do we differentiate management supervision, personal supervision, clinical supervision? There tend to be overlaps but certain professions have developed particular areas of emphasis. Counselling has brought a challenge to clinical and management supervision, demonstrating the importance of some emphasis on the process and personal content of the working relationship.

'You do feel strongly on this, don't you, Alan? I can sense your passion.'

'I have seen too many people burn out because of not having appropriate support, partly because it was not offered, but partly because people do not appreciate what could be helpful, or think it is a sign of weakness.' Alan smiled, he felt better getting that off his chest. 'Thanks for listening, Jan. Let's get back to Dave and Linda.'

Jan felt Alan had said what he needed. She agreed he should use personal therapy to explore issues directly present within himself and supervision for relational issues with clients. She agreed with what he had said as well about people not understanding the importance and value of supervision. 'OK, so back to Dave and Linda. I am wondering if there is anything else you want to explore about your work with Dave? Are they coming back as a couple?'

'They wanted to keep it open for a future time, but for now Dave will continue to come weekly. That is what they wanted and it felt right. Maybe Linda may decide to seek some kind of counselling to help her make sense of her past and how it has affected her, but at the moment she is not looking for this. She may change, it must have been a powerful experience for her in that last session. I will continue to work with Dave, be there for him as he ... well, who knows where it will take him. But I was encouraged by that sense of calm he found during that pit experience. And the fact that I was drawn to that spiritual passage at the end of the last session. There's something deep to Dave. Whilst I am concerned for his wellbeing I also have a sense that somehow he will be OK. I hope I'm right.'

'Maybe it is important to acknowledge that depth that you sense as well.'

'You know I see life as a bit of a journey down a river, or rather we are the river. Sometimes it is smooth, we are smooth, sometimes it, and we, are a raging torrent. Sometimes there are rapids and waterfalls. Dave is going through some rapids, but there is a stillness or calmness, to use his word. Yet it is not an aspect of himself he is familiar with. But he glimpsed it in that session and I am sure it has made a deep impression, I know it did. It's like he has sensed a possibility within himself and I don't think it will go away. I often see clients yearning for some kind of peace, but they provoke chaos because that is what they have been conditioned into from an early age. They often have a dim sense of wanting change, but of not being sure exactly what they want. I think Dave has sensed something in himself that is essentially calm and maybe that will become a more present aspect of his nature in the future.'

How many times had he, Alan, heard clients say how they yearned for some peace, that they were getting too old for the drinking, or they just wanted to settle down, but couldn't get away from old habits. He recognised the conflicts within Dave, the different 'voices' from the different elements within his self-structure. They were all part of Dave but he knew that for the drinking to be brought under control, Dave would have to recreate his sense of self, rebalance the elements that made him who he was and probably introduce some new ones. These could not be forced, it was for them to develop within Dave in response to the experience of being in a warm and unconditionally accepting relationship, as he came to know himself more clearly in response to communicated and heard empathic responses and the experience of entering into therapeutic relationship with someone seeking to be congruent.

Points for discussion

- How effective was Jan in maintaining person-centred values and attitudes in this supervision session, and where do you feel she moved away from this?
- How much knowledge does a supervisor need to have about alcohol and its effects to work effectively with a counsellor such as Alan? What is your level of knowledge and how do you feel about supervising a counsellor working in this area?
- It is possible that Jan and Alan should have explored assumptions further here. Maybe later an assumption was being made by them that Dave was not likely to enter into a suicidal state.
- How would you define and differentiate counselling, management and clinical supervision?
- Where do you distinguish supervision issues from personal therapy issues?
- How would you define intuition and what role does it have in supervision?
- What is the theoretical basis for raising issues (such as Dave's mood) only when they are present in the 'here and now' of the therapeutic relationship?

CHAPTER 4

Supervising the counselling of a sexually abused client*

Jennifer is a client of Laura who is offering private counselling at her home. Jennifer has attended 32 sessions over an 11-month period and had originally started the counselling because she was feeling depressed and life just felt like one huge struggle. By the 33rd session she was beginning to feel ready to work towards an ending. During that session she talked of a trip to visit her sister, and her niece. At that moment she found herself shivering, feeling cold and going silent. She did not know why. She then momentarily passed out during the session and had to be gently awoken by Laura. She spoke of being in her body, looking out but somehow not really seeing anything. In the supervision that followed Laura explored with her supervisor, Malcolm, what might be happening and her sense that something was wrong but she could not define what it was.

Much of the next session was spent talking about the trip to Devon. Jennifer made a reference to the previous session and that it still made her shiver, but she felt OK now. It left Laura unsure, it didn't feel quite right, somehow. She checked it out, but Jennifer confirmed that she was OK. In fact Jennifer's heart was thumping and she knew it was not OK, but she didn't feel able to say it.

The following session, the 35th, began with Laura feeling distinctly disconnected from Jennifer. There was a long silence during which Jennifer had lost all track of time. She later described physical sensations, from below her solar plexus up above her heart, like 'hot gravel grating'. She then talked about her drinking and how it seemed associated with the period when she got home from work and was cooking. She explored this in relation to the effect on her appetite.

There then followed a supervision session in which the possibility of dissociated states emerging was discussed, along with what arrangements might need to be made if Jennifer felt she might want support whilst Laura was away on holiday. It was decided to offer her Malcolm's number if she wished for it.

The following session, the 36th, saw Jennifer connecting with a part of herself that declared that she was seven, but nearly eight years old. Jennifer heard what she was saying, describing being at home, looking out of the window, waiting for

---

*Taken from *Counselling a Survivor of Child Sexual Abuse: a person-centred dialogue* (2003) by Richard Bryant-Jefferies. Radcliffe Medical Press, Oxford.

her father to come home and feeling terrified but not knowing why. She also talked about her dolls, and that she had a secret but she couldn't tell her (Laura) what it was. When she came out of it Jennifer was very emotional, feeling very raw and torn apart, suddenly realising she did not know whether she had had the happy childhood she thought she had had.

Jennifer expresses concern that she was feeling so distressed at a time when Laura was going to be away, and she too was going to have a holiday, making it some weeks before the next appointment. In response to Laura asking what she felt she needed, Jennifer said that having someone she could make contact with if she needed to would help, and preferably someone who would understand and she didn't have to go through everything with. It was at this point that Malcolm was suggested and his number given to Jennifer.

The following dialogue is taken from Laura's next supervision session with Malcolm.

Supervision session

Supervisor: Malcolm

Supervisee/Counsellor: Laura

Client: Jennifer

'Before I say anything about any of my other clients, I do want to mention Jennifer. I gave her your number as we agreed, and she was very grateful. I have only seen her once since our last session, she is currently on holiday and due back next week. I want to bring you up-to-date with the last session.'

'Fine. What's been happening and how are you with the process?'

'In the last session Jennifer twice slipped back into a place in herself that was very much part of her childhood. Firstly she was looking out of the window and said that the window changed to the one she remembered looking out of as a child, and of feeling fear, in fact I think she used the word terror. She had been talking about the evenings and waiting for her partner, Ian to come home. That's a difficult time for her, and she does often drink wine at that time. Oh, and she talked about having disturbed nights, waking up sweaty and uneasy and having to go to another room to calm down. But the window experience seemed to touch some depth. It really seemed to have taken her back, and she talked of being fearful as she looked out, as if she was anticipating something, but she couldn't get hold of what it was.'

'How was that for you?'

'It felt very profound, and very real, and it drew me into a heightened sense of focus. I did have a sense of Jennifer shifting. The silence was intense. It didn't last very long, but it clearly had a powerful effect, and I am sure it was a kind of precursor to what happened later in the session.'

'A powerful effect and then something else happened?'

'Jennifer suddenly started to get very small on me, you know, shift of perspective, and then she began to speak but this time her voice was like a little girl's. She was timid and said she had a secret that she couldn't tell me. She said she knew who I was. I asked her her age, but I didn't push her on the secret. I didn't want her to back away. It seemed right to keep it gentle and non-invasive.'

Malcolm nodded. 'Yes, I think you were very wise. That part of her needs to feel safe with you in order to find its voice in your presence.' He well recognised the need for a slowly, slowly, softly, softly approach.

'Well, she spoke for a while, then flipped into talking about her three dolls, what were they, Lucy, Mandy and Annabelle, and then announced that she had to go. With that she kind of faded and Jennifer in her adult state returned, blinking and bemused, but aware of the conversation that I had had with her child-self, or whatever we should call that part of her that spoke.'

Laura has neglected to remember that Annabelle was the favourite and why. This could be a lapse of memory, but it could be that Laura did not really hear this part, and may indicate that there is something from her own past blocking her.

Unless Malcolm experiences a sense of something important being unsaid, it is unlikely that he will pick up on this. The supervisor needs to be both empathically sensitive and also highly sensitive to his own responses. Offering supervision in a person-centred way requires a somewhat disciplined ability to be open in two directions at the same time as well as attempting to be open to the possibility that things are not being communicated about the client as well.

Malcolm felt very touched by the humanity of it all, of the sense of this little girl finding a voice, perhaps after so many years of silence, and of being heard. He wanted to check out how it had affected Laura and also to support her in being welcoming to this part of Jennifer.

'Very touching, very moving. Maybe you were the first person to really listen to that little girl.'

'I had that wonder. It felt so important to listen and not ask too many questions. I felt like I needed to make a relationship with this part of Jennifer. I really had to talk to her as I might do to a child. I mean, she was a child. There was not a sense of the adult Jennifer in the room.' Laura could feel her own eyes watering as she took herself back to the encounter. 'You know, I wonder why I didn't think of giving her a hug? I guess it was too soon. I mean, I know Jennifer and I would not have a problem with hugging in her adult state, but you know it never crossed my mind to reach out to Jennifer as the seven-year old. I guess it would not have been appropriate, but thinking back now I have this real sense of her needing a hug, somehow, of some kind of reassurance that all will be OK.'

'You look surprised with yourself.'

'I am, and I feel that to have thought about and decided it was inappropriate to offer a hug would be one thing, but to simply not think about it at all is something else. I am feeling very affected as I sit here now, but somehow I wasn't feeling so affected at the time.'

'Any reflections on that?'

'I rather think I was getting caught up in the head and heart, or rather thoughts and feelings split that Jennifer mentioned afterwards, when she talked about knowing and feeling in relation to her changed view of her childhood. She was very shaken and upset when she began to realise that her view of her childhood as being happy may not be true. She talked of realising in her head that this was so, but was struggling to feel it. I think I got stuck in my head somehow, somewhere with Jennifer as a little girl. But then, I do remember feeling I was relating to her as I would a child. I remember noticing that in myself.'

'Stuck in your head.'

'I don't think I was as in touch with feelings as I thought I was, looking back. And yet, thinking about it, I'm not sure how much feeling Jennifer as a child was expressing in that encounter. Let me think back a moment.' Laura took herself back. 'She was afraid, she had a secret but couldn't, no, mustn't tell me because it would get her into trouble. She said her age and that she didn't have anyone to really talk to. It all sounded very matter of fact. And then she brightened and talked about her dolls. Did I miss something? Did I hold back? Was I in a place in myself that was going to be helpful for her? I'm wondering now.'

'Lots of questions ...'

'Yes, I really am wondering if I could have or should have been different. But maybe it was how it has to be for that first encounter. She may not find it hard to trust people. One thing that does strike me is a sense of how she controlled what she said and what we talked about. Yes, now that I think back to it that feels very clear. But that is surely understandable. This is a very frightened part of her that has things she really wants to talk about, but wasn't able to. And she's carrying a secret.' Laura shivered. 'I do need to gain her trust and maybe I must trust how it is developing. I don't feel I did anything out of place. We have only just met.' Laura thought for a moment. 'You know, if Jennifer was aware of what was said during the encounter with her seven-year old sense of self, I wonder if the seven-year old is aware of the conversations Jennifer and I have had when she has been very much her adult self?'

'You wonder who knows what?'

'Something like that. But anyway, I know I need to be attentive to Jennifer the adult who is having to come to terms with her past, and Jennifer the little girl who I hope will feel able to come back again and talk some more. The more I think about it, the more it feels OK, and it is going to take time. And the hug concern does not feel such an issue anymore. But it does all leave Jennifer rather vulnerable, I think, and so she may call.'

Malcolm nodded. There was something nagging away at him, and he couldn't put it aside. Somehow when Laura had spoken about those dolls, it had seemed rather abrupt. Why had she mentioned the dolls? What did they mean?

'There's something troubling me, maybe more nagging at me, and it won't go away. You mentioned the three dolls, and somehow that seemed to get left hanging. Was that how it was, are we mirroring what Jennifer told you, or is there more to it? I'm just struck by the wonder of why did she introduce the dolls?'

Malcolm has used his own experiencing to draw attention to an aspect of what Laura has been describing that he feels troubled by, though he does not know what it is. But he is open and sensitive enough to his own experience to be able to sense the presence of this nagging question. Much that is valuable in supervision can emerge from this kind of processing. The supervisor is reliant on what the supervisee tells him, and often it is only his own internal experiencing that can be used to register when something does not feel right, or is missing, or just doesn't quite add up.

The dolls. Laura thought back. 'Oh yes, I didn't mention it. She said Annabelle was her favourite, yes, her favourite because she was like her and needed to be cared for. How could I have not mentioned that? Oh and she liked dressing her up.'

'You forgot it?'

'Completely. Is that parallel-processing or my stuff? Why didn't I recall it?' Laura thought about it and she had no answer. 'It isn't that I didn't hear it, but after she had said it that part of her had gone.'

'So, my guess is that she was trying to tell you something, and the dolls were maybe a kind of metaphor, or more than a metaphor, for her own experience, perhaps? I'm being tentative here, I don't really want to try and interpret it, but she was I am sure trying to tell you something. The question is, did she feel heard?'

Laura looked and felt uncertain. 'I don't know. Maybe I missed it.' She thought back. 'No, I responded, and it was after my response, yes, immediately after my response, that she faded out.'

'Can you remember what you said?'

'Something like, "Annabelle is rather like you; she needs to be cared for, and you like dressing her up".'

'So it may be that she didn't feel heard and retreated, though it sounds like you did empathise with her quite accurately. So maybe she did feel heard and felt she had said enough at that time. Or maybe some other part of her thought she had said too much and stepped in and blocked her from saying more.'

'I need to think about why I forgot it here, though. It's important. She's telling me she needs to be cared for and I don't know that I really responded directly enough to that. I need to think about that. I wonder if I was reacting out of my own stuff? Silly question, of course I was, what else can I react out of other than myself!' Laura thought back to her own childhood. 'I had a reasonable childhood, a mixture of good and not so good. Did I feel cared for? Sometimes, but not always.'

'You may not necessarily be responding out of your own stuff from the past, of course.'

She smiled to herself. 'You know me too well, thank goodness. The moment you said that my thoughts went to Ian [Jennifer's partner], how much Jennifer needs him to care for her at the moment, and how much she doesn't want to think about the possibility of him not caring. My own sensitivity towards my own need to be cared for I think stopped me fully appreciating the power of what Jennifer was saying. I need to be more aware of that. Yes, that was really helpful.'

When a supervisee appears to miss something when a client is discussing child issues it is easy to assume that the reason is something to do with the supervisee's childhood. As in this case, it may be something much more in the present and it is good practice that Malcolm is open to this and broadens Laura's focus to include considering what is more in Laura's present.

'Is there anything more you feel you need to know, as I don't feel I have much more to say, and there are some other issues with a couple of my other clients I want to mention.'

Malcolm gave himself a moment to check out his own thoughts and feelings about what Laura had been telling him. He felt he had an appreciation of the situation. He thought Laura was doing what needed to be done and that time would tell if memories were going to emerge either through what the seven-year old Jennifer says or through other experiences when Jennifer was in her adult sense of self.

'No, I think that is OK. I think Jennifer has come a long way in the last few sessions and you have been there for her and with her during some difficult experiences. I'm sure you also need your break as well, and give yourself time to really experience yourself in your own world. We spend so much time exposed to our client's inner worlds – we really do need time to be in our own as well! So, I shall be ready if she calls to listen and we'll see what emerges. Like you, I will want to trust the pace of her own process.'

Malcolm ended by asking Laura when she would be back and agreed to call her to let her know whether Jennifer had called, or not. He said that he would agree with Jennifer if she called what he would pass on or whether he would leave it for her to tell Laura herself.

Telephone conversation

Jennifer had been back from her holiday for a week. She had enjoyed her time away but had still felt disturbed. The restless nights, and the urge to drink in the evenings remained present, and she had begun to find herself losing interest in sex with her partner. He had been quite understanding, and she was relieved that it had not caused problems, but it wasn't making life easy, particularly as they had previously discussed and agreed to starting a family.

She had been looking at Malcolm's 'phone number for a couple of days now, trying to decide whether or not to call. To begin with she had found it easy to decide not to, thinking that she would be troubling him and that she could wait for Laura to return. But she had had a particularly difficult night last night, three times she had woken up in a panic, sweating profusely, her heart pounding, and she had really struggled to calm down. She had briefly wondered if she was going mad, and she felt unable to say much to Ian. She couldn't really explain why, she just felt it was difficult somehow. She was again looking at the 'phone number. It was early evening. She had not had a drink but knew she was feeling sorely tempted. Ian wasn't home yet, and wasn't due back for a while. She felt wretched. She didn't know what to do. Two more weeks until she saw Laura seemed an age away.

She closed her eyes and took a deep breath, seeking to steady herself. She felt very shaky inside. Laura had told her that Malcolm was aware of the situation and that he was happy for her to call if need be. And she had said that he took calls around this time each day. It's no good, she thought to herself, I have to 'phone. I cannot go on like this. I have to talk to someone. I have to . . . She wasn't sure what she needed although something about reassurance was around for her.

She picked up the receiver and punched out the numbers on the slip of paper. She heard the pulses and the 'phone began to ring. She could feel her heart pounding as she waited for the receiver to be picked up.

'Hello, Malcolm here.'

'Oh, er, hello, um, my name's, um, Jennifer. Laura mentioned me to you? She said I might 'phone?'

'Yes, yes she did. Hello Jennifer. How can I help?'

'Have you time right now for me to talk?' Jennifer could feel so much tension within her as she asked this question, praying that he would say yes.

'Yes, I have. What's troubling you, Jennifer?' Malcolm could hear the trembling and anxiety in Jennifer's voice.

'Oh I feel awful.' Jennifer let out a long breath, swallowed, and breathed in deeply. 'Since I've been back from holiday, about a week now, I don't know, things seem to be getting worse. I had a terrible night last night. My sleeping is really bad. I wake up with my heart thumping, feeling terrible. I feel I'm going mad. I just need to talk to someone, and, well, I would normally talk to Laura and she's away. So, oh God, am I making any sense? I feel at the end of my tether.'

'Yes, you are making sense but you feel it is driving you mad, at the end of your tether.'

'Yes.' Silence. 'Yes, I feel so wound up with it all, and I don't know what to do or what is happening.'

'Mhmm. Sounds desperate, I really hear the desperation in your voice, Jennifer.' Malcolm was aware that it might well turn into a telephone counselling session and he wanted to be sure that this was what Jennifer wanted. He didn't want to encourage this by his empathic responding unless he was sure that this was what she was seeking. 'And I guess I want to check out what you want from me now, whether you are looking for a telephone counselling session, or if you feel you need to unload.'

'I don't know, I just feel I need to talk to someone who will understand or at least help me make sense of it all, even just a part of it. How long can you give me?'

Malcolm looked at the clock. He could offer Jennifer 20 minutes as he knew he would need some time for himself to process the conversation with Jennifer before his next session.

'20 minutes. Will that be OK?'

'Yes. I may not need that long, but I need to talk. Thank you.' Jennifer paused for a moment before continuing. Somehow she already felt a little easier, although she wasn't at all sure exactly why.

'So, I was hearing the desperation in your voice.'

'Yes, well, I feel I'm bottling things up and it's putting me under pressure. Let me tell you what has been happening and maybe that will help. Is that OK?'

'OK by me, please talk about whatever you feel you need to.' Malcolm genuinely meant this as he said it. He didn't know what Jennifer needed to talk about and felt sure that she would know, even though she might take a while to get to it.

Jennifer noted how genuine that had sounded. 'Well, the holiday – I found myself each evening drinking, and drinking more than I usually do, not just a bottle of wine with the meal, but there would be apéritifs and we would often spend time in the bar in the evening. I got a bit out of order a few times, I got argumentative with Ian, my partner, and, well, I can't remember it all that clearly. I drank far too much the last night and apparently made something of a scene, and, oh I don't know, ended up having a blazing row with Ian. I can't really remember what happened but the flight back, well, we didn't speak very much. I know I had a few more drinks, and since we've been back I've really struggled. And I've really had to fight against the urge to drink more. You know I had a drink problem in the past?'

'Yes, Laura had mentioned that.'

'OK, well, I'm afraid that it will get out of control again, and mess up my relation-ship, and all at a time when we had begun to seriously start to talk about start-ing a family.' With this Malcolm could hear the sound of sobbing down the 'phone.

'I really hear that fear, Jennifer, so much that you don't want to mess up ...' He deliberately left his response open, waiting to hear what Jennifer would choose to focus on.

'I've been so happy and now I feel so wretched.' The sobs became more frequent and Jennifer could feel the tears running down her face. 'I need to get a tissue. Just a minute.'

Malcolm waited. It seemed like an age. Thoughts passed through his mind. Was she OK? Had she switched into a dissociated silence? Might she open herself to feelings that she could not control? Would she be on her own the rest of the evening and how would she cope? He closed his eyes and re-focused himself, recognising that his thinking was running away with itself. Now, let's be calm about this, he said to himself. I need to be here to listen to what Jennifer wants to say, and if I still feel concerned I can ask some of these questions later if they persist and feel relevant. He waited, and heard the 'phone being picked up.

He heard Jennifer breathing out heavily. 'I think I needed that, needed to release some of those tears. I am so afraid of losing it.'

'So afraid of losing what you have.'

'Yes. I need to make sense of what is happening. But I can't, I just know that something doesn't feel right within me. The waking up, the dreams. I don't usually dream, or at least, I don't seem to remember them very clearly. But now, well, now I am getting a sense of what some of them are about, and they always seem to involve me feeling trapped, unable to get away from something, or someone. I wake up sometimes with what feels like a huge pressure on my chest, but I guess that's my heart pounding.'

'So you can't relax, but you are having dreams that you are kind of remembering a little about, and they involve feeling trapped, unable to get away, a feeling of pressure on your body.'

Malcolm was very mindful of the discussions he had had with Laura as to what might be behind what Jennifer was experiencing, but he knew he was there to listen and allow Jennifer to explore and make her own sense of her experience. His sense, though, was that experiences were coming to the surface through the dreaming process and the sense that she had had of pressure on her chest made him think that further, clearer imagery, could be very close. He wondered when Laura was next seeing Jennifer as he could feel his concern as to whether she might experience some flashbacks before then and need support. But he also didn't want to alarm Jennifer or put ideas into her head as to anything that might be behind her experiences. He knew that when he had said 'pressure on your body', he may have overstepped the mark. She had said 'pressure on my chest'. His response had in a way extended what was being described and might push Jennifer towards something she was not yet ready to recognise, this all assuming that some form of sexual abuse lay behind Jennifer's current difficulties. He realised that he needed to explore this in his own supervision.

There was no response from Jennifer. Malcolm could feel the silence incredibly acutely. He remembered how Laura had described the way that Jennifer could flip back into that child-like self, and had passed out completely on one occasion. 'Jennifer,' he said softly, 'I am still here if there is something more that you want to say'.

The silence continued. Jennifer was conscious, but she was miles away from the 'phone conversation, well actually years away, in her past. She did hear Malcolm's voice, but it had seemed very distant. She wasn't really remembering anything specific, though, but it was as though she was held in suspension, not really thinking or feeling, just sitting. She felt small, very small. She became aware that she was rocking gently forwards and backwards, forwards and backwards, again and again and again. This wasn't just a memory, she was aware that this was what she was doing as she sat there, holding the 'phone. She could hear Malcolm's voice, this time it sounded quite urgent. 'Jennifer, are you OK, can you let me know if you can hear me?'

'Yes, yes, I can. Sorry. I ... I'm not sure what happened. I just ... I don't know. I heard your voice just now, you sounded really concerned and I remember hearing you say you were there if there was something else I wanted to say.'

'How are you now, Jennifer?'

'Not sure. Numb. I feel quite ... numb, it's the only word that comes to mind. I somehow feel much calmer. I don't understand.'

'Numb, as though what you had been feeling has somehow been, well, kind of taken away?'

'Yes, like it feels distant. But that can't be. I mean, I ... But I do feel different but I don't feel right. I don't feel me. It's like I feel kind of drugged somehow. As though, as though part of me is missing but I know it isn't really?'

'Part of you is missing but it isn't really.' Malcolm responded directly to the last part of what Jennifer had said.

'Yes. What were we talking about before this happened?'

Malcolm felt his jaw tighten. He knew it had been that comment about pressure on her body. He didn't want to lead her, but then saying those words had clearly had a profound effect on Jennifer, and he had to trust the process here. No sense in being anything other than authentic.

'You were talking about how you felt when you woke up after the disturbing dreams you had been having and I said something like "you are remembering the dreams involve feeling trapped, unable to get away, feeling of pressure on your body".'

'Yes, not feeling able to breathe, I get that.' Jennifer was aware of somehow feeling distant from her dreams though, distant from those feelings. She shook her head and noticed that time had passed, almost 15 minutes since she had started the call. 'I think I flipped back into that place in myself that I have been in with Laura. It all feels so weird and yet somehow I feel easier having just had that experience and talking to you. I think that it had all built up and I needed to let the pressure out. I really appreciate you listening and letting me talk and be silent.'

Sometimes people just need a little time to release thoughts and feelings, and to experience someone else listening and giving them quality attention. When a sense of feeling overwhelmed arises it can leave people with all kinds of self-doubts, and experiences can grow out of proportion, fuelled by mounting anxiety. The reassurance of someone listening and taking them seriously can be extremely helpful and help the person to regain control. This was appropriate in this case as the aim was to offer support for Jennifer during Laura's absence, to help her through anything difficult that might arise.

'That's OK. So you feel a little easier now, less bottled up?'

'Yes, yes. I think my head was spinning with it all and I couldn't get it out. And that strange silence seems to have somehow calmed me down too.'

Malcolm was aware that time was passing. 'I'm glad things feel a little easier for you. I am also aware we only have a few more minutes.'

'OK, look, I feel a lot better having talked to you, Malcolm, and I really hope you don't mind me calling, I really am grateful. I know that the time is nearly up.'

'I'm glad you called and that things have eased. Sometimes it is better to take the pressure off a little and no doubt when Laura returns you can explore it more deeply.'

'Yes.' Jennifer paused. 'I want to pay you for your time, is that OK?'

Malcolm gave Jennifer his hourly rate and she agreed to send him a cheque in the post. They also agreed that she could 'phone again if she needed to, and with the same financial arrangement, and that if things felt too much then maybe they could arrange a definite time for a telephone counselling contact. Jennifer was grateful for this idea but felt that maybe she would wait to see how things went and that she hoped she could wait to see Laura. She agreed that she would let Laura know that she had spoken to Malcolm but also agreed that he could talk about the telephone contact with Laura when he next saw her. She felt in herself reassured in knowing that she could call Malcolm if she felt she needed to. It also kind of felt good that he was supervising Laura as well.

The 'phone call ended and Malcolm slowly put down the receiver. That had been an intense session, he was aware that his level of concentration had been really intense. He generally found this when counselling over the 'phone, trying to pick up on the tone of voice and to be in relationship with a client when the only active sense that could be used was hearing. And, of course, this was his first direct contact with Jennifer. He needed a glass of water and time to clear his head. He jotted down his thoughts and reflections and began to get himself ready for his next face-to-face client.

Points for discussion

- Assess Malcolm's quality of empathy, congruence and unconditional positive regard.
- Would you have wanted to have explored further with Laura any of the issues that arose in supervision. If so, which, and why?
- Should the supervisor be the person to be available to a client when the counsellor is away? Discuss the advantages and disadvantages of this arrangement.
- What were your reactions to the telephone conversation?
- Write supervision notes for this session.

CHAPTER 5

Supervising the counselling of a client facing the diagnosis of a progressive disability*

Gerry has been diagnosed as possibly having MS, and is awaiting an appointment with the consultant neurologist. He has been experiencing symptoms of the condition and it has affected his mood. As a result his GP suggested he talk to a counsellor and he has had two sessions of counselling with Maureen. He has struggled to make his feelings visible, but they have emerged, in particular feelings of hopelessness. Maureen has sought to give Gerry time and space to express whatever is present for him. She realises this is a very sensitive and painful time, and Gerry needs to be able to find his own way to make sense of what has happened. He is already fearing his progression into disability. Towards the end of the second session he voices appreciation to Maureen. 'You are steady, someone I can rely on, someone who, I don't know, it's hard to describe, but I do sense that you are listening, really listening, and that feels very important to me at the moment. Sometimes I feel like I'm going mad, but you take me seriously, you listen, you tell me what you hear and what you feel. That feels good, somehow. Like, it sort of feels real? No games.'

Gerry's counsellor Maureen nodded. 'Yeah, no games.' Another moment of connection and a silence. 'None of this is a game.'

Maureen takes her counselling experience with Gerry to her supervision with Donna, with the intention of reflecting on the two counselling sessions they have had so far.

---

* Taken from *Counselling for Progressive Disability: person-centred dialogues* (2004) by Richard Bryant-Jefferies. Radcliffe Medical Press, Oxford.

Supervision session

Supervisor: Donna

Supervisee/Counsellor: Maureen

Client: Gerry

Maureen had been talking about some of her other clients in the supervision session and she wanted to spend some time talking about Gerry and the impact on her of working with him.

'I have another new client at the surgery, referred by the GP. He's experiencing symptoms which he's convinced is MS though he's waiting to see the neurologist. He's getting shooting pains and headaches, blurred vision, his movement isn't good. Seems he is needing space to talk through coming to terms with it and the implication for his future.'

Donna nodded. 'That sounds quite heavy and I notice from your tone of voice that there's suddenly a real seriousness in the atmosphere.'

'Yes, it's a tough one.'

'Seen other clients in this position?'

Maureen shook her head. 'No, not like this, waiting for a diagnosis with a head full of fears that are just, yeah, what you'd feel.'

'So I'm wondering how it is leaving you feeling and what impact that is having on the forming of the therapeutic relationship. How many times have you seen him?'

'Twice. The first session he really struggled to say much about it. There were a lot of feelings present but he was trying to hold them back. But towards the end he became more emotional and talked about his fear of being in a wheelchair. Said that giving his son a bicycle for his birthday recently had brought home to him how limited he was becoming. So many assumptions about his future are evaporating. A lot of loss.'

'Yeah, and I appreciate that hearing you speak about him there is a real sensitivity coming across to me.'

'I really feel for him, for his struggle to make sense of it and to adjust to it all. I know that remission can occur, but for many people the future is one of pain and disability, and he's only in his early 30s. I know people much younger than him develop the condition, but that's no help to Gerry. He has to find his own way through this.'

'Yes, your head knows that remission can occur but your feelings . . . ? I'm aware of not hearing about your feelings?'

The supervisor hasn't heard about the impact on her supervisee's feelings and offers an opportunity to explore this.

'I feel the awesome nature of what he is facing, the huge impact that it is having and will have on his life, you know, I mean, all of his life. I am aware after being with him how much I take my own health for granted in many ways. It's the kind of thing that you think will happen to someone else. You don't think about it in relation to yourself, at least, not unless it is in the family or has affected a close friend and you already have an appreciation of how it can affect people.' Maureen wasn't feeling unduly emotional as she spoke, somehow the hugeness of it all was leaving her feeling, well, she wasn't sure exactly what it was, there was a kind of numbness that sort of seemed linked to the overwhelming nature of it all. She had gone quiet.

'Can feel overwhelming?' Donna was sensing that Maureen was very much in awe of it all. It felt huge.

'It makes me feel somehow quite small. Like where do you begin? I mean, I know I can't make it better, I can't even really offer him hope.'

'It feels hopeless to you?' Donna was interested in pursuing this sense of hopelessness. Was Maureen feeling impoverished, deskilled in some way, she wondered.

'I can only imagine what it must feel like to be faced with something like this.'

Donna nodded, 'it's left to your imagination'.

'And it's hard to connect with what it must feel like.'

'You feel unable to connect with your own feelings?'

An important question, summing up the difficulty that Maureen is facing. It leaves her exploring in her own mind whether this is so. It also opens her to focus on her own experiences in this area, and a memory surfaces as a result.

The room had gone quiet, and both were talking quietly and reflectively. Maureen thought about that last response. Do I feel unable to connect with *my* feelings? She wondered about it. True, she wasn't sure what she felt. She thought about her own family, no one had had MS. She could remember an aunt who had arthritis and had done for many years. She could remember visiting her as a child. Even then she wasn't too mobile. As a child she hadn't really appreciated it, remembered being told off on one occasion for being too boisterous and running into her aunt, which had caused her pain. She'd been told off about it, but she hadn't really understood why. She'd only been about six or seven at the time. Later on she'd begun to understand. But it had eased for a while in her life although now she was quite elderly and being cared for in a nursing home. She realised she hadn't seen her for the longest while and made a mental note to do something about that.

'You seem lost in thoughts, Maureen. Anything in particular?'

Maureen smiled. 'I was back in the past.' She told her about the incident with her aunt and how she now realised she wanted to see her, talk to her, maybe try and understand from her what it had been like facing a progressive disability. 'It's not the same but in her days there weren't the treatments for arthritis that there are today. She has suffered from progressive disability throughout her life. I feel I want to talk to her.'

'Listen to her or say something to her?'

Maureen was back to the incident. She'd felt awful, she'd loved her aunt, and she'd seen her many times later in childhood, but her shriek of pain, she could still hear it. Maureen felt her emotions rising, the tears in her eyes, and they began to seep out and down her cheeks. 'I didn't understand. I didn't mean to hurt her, but I did. They told me off, but I didn't know, I didn't understand.'

Donna sensed the shift and stayed with Maureen. 'You didn't understand, how could you, you were a small child.'

'But they made me think that I should have known, should have understood, should have been more careful.'

'Mhmm, should have known, should have been more careful, but you didn't know.'

'No, I didn't.' Maureen felt the tide of emotion passing, and began to dry her eyes. 'But I needed to.'

'Your need to know sounds quite important to you.'

As Maureen heard Donna she found herself flipping back to Gerry. She shook her head. 'That's it, isn't it? Needed to know, should have known. She hadn't told me about her pain. I should have known. Gerry hasn't really told me about his pain, and again I should know, I need to know. I've got to be careful, here. Stuff from the past, it never lets you go, does it?'

Donna shook her head, 'can leave us with sensitivities however much we work on it.'

'OK. So, I can see my sensitivity, and I need to be aware of that. I need to be open but allow Gerry to go at his pace. The "should know" from the past I have to ignore. That was then, not now. But I do feel I need more knowledge of Gerry's condition generally. Someone suffering from MS isn't something I've worked with a great deal. Maybe I should contact one of the MS networks, get some information. I don't know, I feel I need to know more. And as soon as I hear myself say that, I know as well that in reality I'm working with feelings of loss, or at least potential loss, which I am used to working with.'

'But there is something different about this?'

Maureen nodded. 'Yes.'

'Can you get hold of what that difference is, what it feels like?' Donna was circling her hands in front of her as she spoke. She could feel inside herself an urge to somehow get some clarity, some sense of what it was that Maureen was experiencing.

Part of the last session came back to her, that feeling of awkwardness that had suddenly arisen in her and persisted for a while. 'There were times in the last session when I felt awkward.'

'Awkward?'

The supervisee has moved to a recognition of a particular feeling that has been present for her in the sessions.

'Yes, a kind of uncomfortable awkwardness. It's kind of difficult to describe, but I felt sort of, well ...' She thought about it more, 'well, awkward. But there was more to it than that. It was quite strong, you know, and, yes, really uncomfortable.'

'Mhmm, so something about what was happening was leaving you feeling this way, uncomfortable, awkward, and it persisted.'

'Yes.'

'Can you reconnect with that feeling now rather than think about it?' Donna was aware that there could be a tendency in supervision to talk about feelings when often what was needed was an opportunity to connect with them and allow them to become present and experienced in the session. Often that helped the supervisee to process them.

Maureen sat. She was aware she was thinking about them. 'I'm still in my head, here. I need to get into my body, I think.'

Donna was struck by that comment. 'Need to get into your body. Somehow there's a kind of physiological reaction but you're not in touch with it?' She was mindful that Gerry was bringing an issue concerned with coming to terms with a physical condition.

Maureen sat and brought herself in her imagination to how it had been with Gerry. She allowed herself to be with the issues he had brought, with his upset, his tears, his despair, his needing an answer to that question, 'why me?'. She could feel a knot in her solar plexus, heavy, dark. Her arms felt strangely numb. She stayed with the experience. She felt heavy in the chair, like it was hard to move. She felt tired, she could feel her eyes getting heavy. There was a kind of bleakness to the experience. A real sense of what's the point. That was what Gerry had said, at least, she thought he had.

'What are you feeling, Maureen? You look very serious.' Maureen had her eyes closed and her face seemed quite tense.

> The supervisor offers an opportunity for Maureen to put into words what has become present for her. She is now exploring elements that were present at some level within herself within the session but which, at the time, she was not connected with and which could have affected the quality and nature of her empathy, and certainly her degree of congruence.

'It feels really bleak, and heavy, and a sense of "what's the point?". It feels like I'm surrounded by ..., well, it's like a kind of heavy treacle but it isn't. It's not sticky or anything like that.' She thought about it some more, trying to get a sense of what would describe this feeling, the sensation that was pervading her body. Her mind suddenly thought of how she was sitting on the earth, held down by gravity. She wasn't sure where the image had come from, but it made sense. Yes, gravity. 'I've got it, it feels like gravity has increased, like there's a pull on me, making it difficult to move easily.' She was amazed how heavy she was feeling, yet she knew nothing had changed, not really changed, and yet she felt so heavy, so stuck.

'So there's a real heaviness, like gravity has increased and is sort of pinning you down?'

'Not exactly pinning me down. I know I can move, I know I have that freedom, and yet it's difficult.' She realised she was back to thinking about Gerry. 'I'm back in my head again, thinking about Gerry. The thought has just struck me that as I sit here feeling the heaviness, the difference is that he's in pain, I'm not.'

'Mhmm, he's in pain and you're not.'

'And that . . .' Maureen stopped again, yes that was it, 'yes, I'm not in pain and he is, and I feel uncomfortable about that.'

'So not sharing his pain, or not being in pain, makes it uncomfortable for you to be with him?'

'If I was in pain like him, maybe it would be easier to listen to him. Not sure why I said that.' Maureen had her eyes closed as she sat trying to stay in touch with the experience.

'Mhmm, if you had his pain, then maybe . . .'

Maureen cut into what Donna was saying, 'yes, if I had his pain, yes, that's it. That's the awkwardness.' She opened her eyes and was aware that the heaviness was passing and she was suddenly beginning to feel more alert again. 'Yes, I feel awkward because I'm pain free, he isn't. I feel that I need to be feeling what he is, which I can't. I can only sense his reaction to his pain. It's like, we hear our clients talk about their emotional pain, you know, and we can get a sense of that, sometimes. I mean, we don't actually feel what they feel, but in a way we do, kind of tune in, be somehow in their world, their frame of reference.'

> The supervisee makes a connection. She has realised the roots of the awkwardness that she has felt and has, in effect, integrated the experience more fully into her experience. It will enable her to become more fully and authentically present with her client.

Donna was nodding and listening intently, very aware that Maureen had shifted quite clearly from being heavy and serious looking to being suddenly more alert. She didn't say anything, simply nodded slowly, not wanting to interfere in Maureen's train of thought.

'But this is physical pain as well and I cannot get into that experience. I can get a sense of his despair, his feelings about his pain, and yes, I've had headaches, but . . . oh, I don't know, I cannot get into the pain itself. And that's what feels awkward. Like I cannot get into part of his experience.'

'OK, you can't get into his physical pain, but you can sense and feel something of the nature of his emotional pain.'

'Yes, his fear of the future, his sense of loss, yes, those are present. I can relate to them. I can sense their presence. But the physical pain, no, I've not experienced what he must be going through.'

'You need to experience his pain, or pain like his, to feel you can empathise?'

'I think I do.'

'Mhmm. It has to be his pain?'

'Not sure what you mean, it sounds like you've something in mind.'

'Well, we don't necessarily experience our client's emotional pain, but our emotional reaction to their pain which is then kind of informed by our own experiences of emotional pain. Does that make sense?'

'Yes. So I can hear and appreciate what my client tells me of their emotional pain, using my experience of my own feelings when I am with them and my own experiences in my own life, yes?'

'Is that making sense in relation to your experience?'

'Yes, it does.' Maureen stopped for a moment, thinking about all of this. OK, so I can use my knowledge and experience of pain to get an appreciation for what a client is going through, we have a kind of emotional language, even though I cannot actually really know what my client is feeling from the words they use because they may be attaching a different meaning to the one I do to a particular word. But we have enough to communicate and for me to gain an empathic understanding. 'But I can't get into his physical pain, Donna, I can't get a sense of what it must be like.' She thought back over the sessions. 'I can't remember him really describing the pain, or has he and I've lost it?' She couldn't recall. 'I don't think he has.'

'OK, so he hasn't really talked about it, and you sense a difficulty in actually being able to appreciate what his personal pain is like, and it leaves you with some inner discomfort and an awkwardness.' Donna sought to sum up where they had got to. She was aware that their time was nearly up, but she also sensed that the exploration hadn't ended. But maybe it didn't have an end, it would continue during the time Maureen was working with Gerry. Or maybe it was a simple fact that if you hadn't genuinely experienced a particular physical pain, it was difficult to really empathise with the experience of someone else for whom that pain was a reality.

'I mean, I know pain, the physical pain I've experienced. You don't give birth to children without knowing that, and, yes, I have pain, but it is *my* pain. It's kind of personal to me in some way.'

'Something very personal about pain, your pain is not your client's pain.'

'No. I need to be able to get a sense of his pain.'

'Your need?' Donna was aware of the forcefulness of what Maureen had said.

'Mhmm, that doesn't sound very person-centred, it's my client's needs that are important, but no, I have a need here as well. I need to appreciate more his pain.' She paused. 'I'm not getting in there. I need to get in there, I need to be more open, somehow. I think I'm closed down. It's no good. I need to be affected. Dammit, I want to be affected.'

'You're fired up, Maureen. What's happening for you?'

'Frustration, despair.' She could feel tears welling up. 'Shit. He's a lovely guy, he's got to me. I want to make it better. I can't. Why do people have to suffer like this? I watched a TV programme last night about someone coping with disability, lost the use of their arms and legs. Talking about their struggle to accept their situation, how they fought against accepting it, battled, argued with God, pleaded, but nothing changed, just got worse.'

'Why do people suffer? And you're suffering as you think about it.'

'Makes me so angry. Just doesn't seem fair. Is this it? One life, and the dice is loaded?'

'Strong feelings, Maureen, how the hell do we make sense of it?'

'I guess everyone has their own way, I just haven't found one.'

'What makes it hard to accept it with Gerry?'

'He's a nice guy, just doesn't seem fair. Guess I warmed to him pretty quickly, think I've got too much sympathy and not enough empathy.'

'Mhmm, that's how it feels?'

'But I care. And yet he hasn't really told me that much about his pain.'

'Maybe he isn't ready yet to tell you, Maureen. As you said earlier, it's personal, it's an intimate experience, maybe he's not ready yet to be that personal.'

Maureen took a deep breath. 'You're right, of course. Yes. Yes. But I still want to get in there.'

Donna nodded, 'yes, I hear you, and Gerry must decide what he is going to tell you, and when. But perhaps what we have talked about has left you more open in some way to him, and maybe you'll be different in the next session because of this?'

'I think I will. I do feel different, more alert, more present somehow. Something has shifted in me. More aware of my reactions, of what I feel about it all. Yeah, that feels good. I need this. That's partly why I come, of course?' She smiled.

Maureen acknowledges that a shift in her experiencing of herself has occurred. The comment 'more present, somehow' is significant. She is becoming more open to the range of reactions that have been occurring within her in response to Gerry. She will feel more present because more of her is present to her. This means that there is a higher likelihood that more of her will be emotionally/psychologically present for Gerry which in turn will help more of him to come into the therapeutic relationship.

'Yes, part of the mystery of supervision is how we unravel these kinds of knots through this process. But we shouldn't be surprised. It's similar to what clients do when they talk through issues.'

'I know, but I am grateful for it. I learn so much, and it is a constant exploration of myself. I know we talk about clients, but often it comes down to *me*, *my* reactions, *my* process, how *I'm* affected by the client. It's just such a privilege in many ways to have this space.'

'Yes, and a professional requirement, of course, to ensure that we are safe, the client's safe, and that we are really able to be authentically and empathically present in a warm and accepting relationship with our clients.'

'Thanks, Donna.'

The session drew to a close. Maureen felt ready to work with Gerry, somehow more enlivened, more present and ready to connect with him therapeutically and as a human being. Maureen left feeling nourished and enriched by the experience. She realised she was chasing words to hang on her experience. She let it go. She didn't need words. She knew she was in a different place and it felt like the right place to be. It felt healthy. She felt more alive. She turned on the radio, Mendelssohn's Italian Symphony. She breathed in deeply, allowing the sound to permeate her being. It felt good to be alive. And there was Gerry. What did he need at this moment to feel good to be alive?

Points for discussion

- Assess the supervision session from the standpoint of person-centred theory.
- How has the supervisor used her own inner experience to shape her responses to Maureen?
- What are the feelings that you sense to be present for Maureen as she describes her new client, Gerry? Could there be more feelings other than those she has voiced?
- What expectations would you have if you were referred a client in Gerry's situation before reading this dialogue. Has reading this session changed these expectations?
- Do you feel Donna responded effectively to Maureen's feelings? Would you have responded differently?
- Write supervision notes for this session.

CHAPTER 6

Supervising the counselling of a client with a disability who is in the process of accepting her need to use a wheelchair*

Jim is a counsellor who visits his client, Pauline, at her home. Pauline's disability means she is not very mobile. Jim sees her in her lounge. The seating is such that at first he felt rather distant from Pauline, but has since moved to be physically closer. This was mutually agreed. Sometimes Pauline's partner, Diana, is in the home. For Pauline the issue is a simple one – should she accept that she has to use a wheelchair on a regular basis? She is weighing up the pros and cons and it is linking into a range of feelings and concerns as she does this. Issues addressed include the experience of pain and whether the counsellor can really understand the nature of the pain of another person, the prospect of using a wheelchair, the sense that Pauline has of having a part of herself that accepts the inevitability of the wheelchair – 'accepting me', and an 'anxious me' that is concerned with what it would mean.

Jim has explored his feelings of powerlessness in a previous supervision session. His supervisor, David, also picked up on how Jim was describing Pauline in a very factual way and was wondering what feelings were present.

In the counselling session prior to the supervision session that follows, the client Pauline talks of her need to accept her situation. However, as the session proceeds she engages with strong feelings and a cathartic release occurs in which she talks of her experience of her whole body crying and being in mourning for the loss that it has experienced of mobility and pain-free existence. Jim begins to talk about his experiencing of counselling Pauline.

---

* Taken from *Counselling for Progressive Disability: person-centred dialogues* (2004) by Richard Bryant-Jefferies. Radcliffe Medical Press, Oxford.

Supervision session

Supervisor: David

Supervisee/Counsellor: Jim

Client: Pauline

'I need to spend some time processing my experience with Pauline yesterday, the client who is struggling with whether or not she should use a wheelchair.'

David nodded. 'The way you said that seems to communicate that it was quite powerful. You sounded quite overwhelmed somehow.' David had noted that there was a certain quietness to Jim's voice, as if he had just come through something extremely draining.

'It was overwhelming. Pauline had a major I guess you'd call it cathartic episode. She really connected with something deep, some very body-centred feelings.'

'Body centred?'

'She talked about her whole body wanting to cry, she used some incredibly powerful images, of her skin wanting to ... I can't recall exactly how she said it, but like it wanted to cry, like tears coming through her skin. And she talked of feeling as if she, her body, was in mourning, mourning for the losses, you know, loss of mobility, loss of pain-free existence, I guess, though I don't recall we ever got to anything specific like that. It was more general.'

'So her whole body wanting to cry?'

'And so much emotion, so much seemed to be present for her. She described it as if she had a field of emotion and it was all feeling so much.' Jim could recall vividly now how it had been, sitting with her, holding her arm. He remembered her saying 'oh dear' again and again as the waves of feeling surged through her.

'So much emotion, and how was it for you listening to her, attending to her?'

'I felt quite calm and at the same time felt the enormity of what was happening for Pauline. The way she described it, I hadn't heard someone talk quite that way before. Her whole body in mourning image was so, well, tangible, you know? And, well, it really made sense given that she has got pain in so much of her body. There was something that just felt right about her whole body feeling like that.'

David nodded. 'I'm also aware of feeling the enormity of it and I am hearing about it second hand, as it were. I am aware of what I am feeling listening to you, and that is something about feeling my focus is sharpened up and it makes me feel alert. I am wondering whether that has any relevance to your experience?'

David uses his own experience of his reactions to what Jim is saying to try and inform what else may be present for Jim. This can be a valuable approach in supervision. The supervisor can connect with feelings and

> thoughts that whilst not consciously present for the counsellor, do repre-
> sent something significant for the therapeutic relationship they have with
> their client.

Jim thought about it. 'Yes, I was very much alert, and thinking about it, I was
sitting on the padded stool in that session – I'd moved closer to her in the previous session when she was distressed, and used the stool all through that last
session. Thinking back to it, my body was quite rigid, and I was quite stiff afterwards.' Jim thought about it a bit more. Yes, he really had been focused during
that emotional release, and he remembered what Pauline had said about fields
of emotion. He found himself wondering how that might have affected him.
'I've just remembered something else. Pauline talked of her belief that she had
an emotional field, that emotions weren't simply by-products of chemical reactions. I'm just wondering how, if that's the case, her field of emotion might
impact on my own.'
'Mhmm. So, the focus left you feeling stiff but that could have been the seating
position. You felt focused, alert, and then this notion of a field of emotion
impacting on you.' David was aware of this idea, but he left it open for Jim to
follow up with what was present for him.
'Quite tense as well.' Jim thought for a moment. He wanted to say something
more. 'I do think feeling gets across, I'm sure I pick up on my client's experience
in some way, tune in, particularly in those really deep moments, but maybe it is
happening all the time?'
'Maybe. If true, and I agree that this may be happening, we have to be at least
open to the possibility, then it really does have implications for the nature, purpose, role, impact of therapeutic relationship – both on the client and the
counsellor.'
'Makes me think of just how important those core conditions are, and how we
need to be authentic.' Jim was reflecting back to the experience with Pauline.
He was back with that sense of calmness that had been present for him as well.
'I'm also aware of that calmness, and can feel it being very present as we are
discussing this now.'
'Interesting, that you felt tense and you were also saying you felt calm, and that
calmness is present.'
Jim was nodding thoughtfully. Yes, he had felt calm, he was feeling calm, and yet
... Where was the tension he had felt? He tried to think back to the session.
He could suddenly see Pauline very clearly again talking about feeling her
nerves wanted to cry, yes, that was it, her nerves, her body, her muscles,
her skin wanted to cry. He noted he was taking a deep breath and felt a wave of
sadness within himself. It was quite intense and took him by surprise.
David noted the look of surprise on Jim's face and commented. 'Feelings?'
'I just suddenly went back to something Pauline had said, she'd begun saying,
before talking about her whole body being in mourning, about her nerves
wanting to cry, her muscles wanting to cry, like it was her diseased body
wanting to release so much. And I'm aware I'm in touch with some really

strong feelings of sadness just at the moment.' Jim went back into silence as he felt more the presence of the sadness within him. It felt ... He wasn't sure, but it wasn't a surging sadness, more gentle, calm, but very present, very present. Hard to locate exactly. He was aware his own eyes were watering.

'That sadness is really present for me, David, really present. I need to be with this and see where it leads. But it feels almost as though I'm experiencing some kind of, I don't know, sympathetic reaction to what Pauline experienced. I mean sympathetic in the sense that it feels like ...' He paused again, he knew he wasn't sure how to describe what he was feeling. 'Guess I really made a connection. It's like it just makes so much sense for a person to feel the way Pauline was feeling. But I wonder how many people are that sensitive?'

'Seems that maybe you are, Jim, it really has touched you.'

Rather than empathise with Jim's comment, David brings the focus into Jim's own experience and reaction, into the here and now. By holding Jim in this way, and in effect not allowing him to speculate on the sensitivity of others, he offers opportunity to further explore his reaction. However, Jim isn't there. He's still with his own thoughts and wondering about how others might be carrying similar feelings locked up inside of themselves, locked in their bodies.

Jim continued to sit with the feeling of sadness that had become very present for him. And he was aware that his thoughts were not just focused on Pauline, rather he was thinking about just how many people must have this kind of reality which hasn't broken into their awareness, how many people are in a sense walking around in bodies that are crying out, but aren't heard? Yet at the same time, Jim was thinking that it was such a weird way of thinking about things, and part of him felt that it was too way-out. And yet ... another deep breath and he began to speak, but not before he had shaken his head a few times. 'I guess that in a way I've been put in touch with my own bodily awareness to some degree, and yet I have nothing to compare to Pauline. But it does leave me wondering, you know, just what may be present within our bodily experience which somehow does not reach consciousness. And what that's all about.' Jim noted that the sadness was lifting, that he was beginning to feel ... the only word that made any sense was 'liberated' from what he had been experiencing. Then he realised that, of course, for someone like Pauline there was unlikely to be any liberation, not in life anyway. He pursed his lips. 'I'm beginning to wonder how this may all be affecting my empathy, David.'

'That these feelings could be affecting how you empathise?'

'I didn't feel blocked in the session and so maybe it is just where I am in myself now, but I realise that we never really got into what her body was really mourning for. There was just this cathartic release.'

'You sound like you feel that there should have been more insight?'

Hearing David put it like that, Jim knew instinctively that his response was 'no'. 'It's not like that. No, I mean, I guess I'd have been interested to know, yes, that's it, I'm sure it's my own curiosity, but it wasn't something Pauline got into, and we were heading towards the end of the session anyway. But that's my need to know. Maybe at some level Pauline does know, perhaps she is very aware and chose not to go down that route.' Jim felt sure that it was his curiosity and he was mindful that whilst that was a good quality for a counsellor, it could become extreme and be simply just plain nosy. He didn't feel it was that, more he felt he needed to connect with what was happening for Pauline. It intrigued him. He glanced at the clock and was aware that the supervision session was passing. And he had other matters he wanted to raise.

It is fascinating how much can arise from counselling. So much time could be spent in supervision processing it, and yet there is a time-constraint to this. Whilst one has to be practical, the truth is that generally speaking one could always use more supervision time to explore the counselling process, the impact on the counsellor, the effect of the counsellor's responses on the client and the experience of bringing the session's therapeutic content into the supervisory relationship.

'I'm feeling clearer, it's been good to air this and speculate a bit, and I can recognise and own my curiosity, and that may help me allow Pauline to choose her own focus next session.'

'That's important, don't forget, she will have a week to live with that experience as well, and it will have been more real, more pertinent for her than for you, and she will make of it what she will. She needs to be allowed the freedom to make her own sense of it and to integrate the experience and the meaning she attaches to it. It sounds incredibly profound and I am sure it has had, and is having, a significant impact on her. But what that will be, who knows?'

'I know that I don't know. But I'm so glad it happened.' Jim paused. 'I also wanted to just highlight another thing that emerged during the sessions, I think it was the previous one. There was something about Pauline experiencing anxiety about the possibility of having to accept using a wheelchair, and what it would mean. She really does fear losing her own mobility so much, and I can appreciate that. And she also spoke of an acceptance as well?'

'Acceptance? Of being in a wheelchair?'

'Sort of. She said something about it being quite a calm place inside herself, a sort of place where it was OK, but that her sense was that her anxiety kept her away from that place that it was somehow dangerous? She didn't say that, it's my own impression as I sit here now and talk about it.'

'Like it's dangerous to accept it?'

'Like it's OK to accept it but there is a danger in allowing that acceptance to dominate. It's like her anxious self wants to keep her independent and on her own two feet at virtually any cost.'

'Which is very often the response in these situations.'

'And she recognises this. She sees it as a battle and each time she has to give something up it is like a retreat ready to kind of re-group to fight to cope at the next level of disability. But I guess I was struck by this struggle between the two and how she could sense this calm acceptance but ... oh yes, I think she said something about when she finds that place then it triggers the anxiety again.'

'Like the anxiety becomes a reaction to, or against, acceptance?'

'That's right. In a way it was confusing and I guess I wanted to talk it out, try to order it in my own head because I'm sure we will come back to this. The notion that the structure of self is composed of "configurations" (Mearns, 2000) well, I'm sure it has application.' Another thought was with Jim. 'As I say this I am struck by the sense that at some level, or in some part of herself, Pauline knows that it will be OK to use a wheelchair. But to this other part of her structure of self that is so dangerous.'

'So there is something about this other part, possibly her anxious part though not necessarily, that presumably feels very threatened, very threatened, and gives Pauline an experience to take her away from it.'

'From what is threatening her?'

'Maybe, but it could be something that is simply threatening to that part of her self.'

'Like the part of her that, for instance, might want to preserve independence or feel in control.'

'Could be. Could be all kinds of things and obviously whilst we can speculate we cannot bring this into the session and start trying to hypothesise as to what parts exist.'

'I know. These parts are very much the client's experience and it is for Pauline to identify what they are through her own, I guess, self-experience.' Jim thought for a moment. 'The prospect of being in a wheelchair must challenge so many beliefs, notions, concepts that a person has about themselves. I'm struck as I sit here by the enormity of it. I mean, I kind of knew it at a sort of intellectual level and had a sense of the emotional impact it has on people, but it absolutely, well, it's like almost throwing a hand grenade into someone's structure of self. It's mind blowing.'

David was nodding. He hadn't quite thought of it this way, and found himself responding, 'literally – and emotions too.'

They both lapsed into silence each, in their own way, having connected with something that was suddenly very real, very present and very awesome.

In supervision it can be important to, in a very real sense, honour the client for what they are going through. Sometimes the recounting of sessions, the therapeutic speculation, the exploration of the quality and nature of the therapeutic relationship is called to a halt by a moment of respectful silence for a client. Holding this kind of respectful silence, acknowledging the immensity of what a client is passing through, is important. In our busy, busy world we can lose sight of the need for this time, rushing on to talk about the next client. Counsellors, and supervisors, need to share silences when they arise in the context of their exploration of the work being done with a client. Taking time to be with what, as in this case, has become suddenly very real, very present and very awesome.

It was Jim who broke the silence. 'And it makes me think of how many people come through this experience, adapt, adjust and emotionally and mentally survive and in fact grow through it. And I guess many do not as well.'

David was thinking of the Chinese glyph for, what was it, crisis. He'd read about it years ago, that it was composed of two other glyphs; one for danger, the other for opportunity. Seemed to sum it up. He shared his remembering with Jim.

Jim responded. 'Yes, I'd come across that. And it does have a lot of meaning for these kinds of situations. But it isn't just mobility that is in danger in Pauline's mind, it is the different parts of her sense of self, or that make up her sense of self, which are being threatened or challenged. I'm kind of tempted to say that she knows it won't stop her mobility, but it will affect her independence if her leg muscles weaken, or even her joints may stiffen from reduced usage, and that's a big fear for her.'

'Yes, and there is also the fact of how she will feel being viewed as a person in a wheelchair rather than standing upright.'

'Fear of the "does she take sugar" syndrome?'

'Partly that, but what it means to her as, well, as a woman. There are going to be so many aspects of all of this that she may want or need to work on. It could be really long-term work, you know, if that is what Pauline wants.'

'Time will tell on that. My sense is that she may, but then she may, if she gets to the point of deciding to accept the wheelchair, decide that that's enough. She's come to terms with it enough to get on with her life.'

'And we must trust her in that, she will know her needs and what is uppermost for her.'

Jim thought for a moment. 'We can "over-therapise" can't we? We can get so caught up in all the emotional implications, and helping a client untangle or get clarity about their structure of self that we can forget that perhaps the client simply wants to have space to come to a decision and, having made their decision, move on and make the best of it, whatever it might be.'

'We have to be ready to accept that, but also aware that for some people they will want to work more deeply and extensively, and so we offer them that. But as a person-centred therapist you/we are not going to push them either way, of course.'

'No, but you can appreciate the temptation to cling to clients and in effect push them on a psychological journey that is the desire of the therapist more than that of the client.'

'And that has to be watched for and, well, hopefully supervision will pick that up.'

'You know, I think more and more people are wary of that. I think there is a more goal-oriented sense among people these days. They have a problem, they want it sorted.'

'But often they want relief of symptoms, and they can get that, with a short period of counselling, maybe, or prescribed medication . . .'

'Or something more illicit, or, of course, alcohol.'

'. . . but it takes time to really adjust to these kinds of life changes, like Pauline is facing, and to do so in a way that is healthy for her structure of self. It puts it under a lot of strain, and yet, as we know, it can be the making, or prove the breaking, of people.'

'Yeah.' He thought of Pauline. Her sense was that she was a fighter, that whatever happened, she would continue being herself, even if she had to go around on wheels. In a funny kind of way, he suddenly got the sense that it might make her even more formidable – no longer so drained by the constant physical, and emotional and mental struggle to keep mobile, and able to move around more easily. But she had a huge adjustment to make. He wanted to help her in that, if that was her choice. He kind of felt it would be, but he knew that it was up to her. There was an inevitability about it, simply more a matter of time, of when rather than if. When the time is right for her, when she is ready to embrace change – or was it truer to say when change embraced her?

> The moment, when such change arrives, will be a 'turning point'. Such a moment has been described in the *I Ching*: 'There is movement but it is not brought about by force . . . The movement is natural, arising spontaneously. For this reason the transformation of the old becomes easy. The old is discarded and the new is introduced. Both measures accord with the time; therefore no harm results' (Wilhelm, 1968, p. 97).

Jim was left feeling a huge sense of respect for Pauline. And as he connected with that feeling he remembered that moment the session before last where their eyes had met, that moment of real, deep, calm connection. He described it to David.

'Made a deep impression on you, felt calm, you say?'

'Very calm, very steady, a real moment of meeting, you know?'

'And I just wonder how important that moment was for what followed in the next session. Maybe there was something communicated in that moment that allowed her feelings – the emotions, that sense of her body wanting to cry – to happen in your presence.' David smiled. 'I'm really touched by the work you are doing, Jim, and I have a real sense of how connected you are. I guess, and I'm putting a supervisor hat on here, I guess I need to say keep space for yourself. And I am aware that it is a need to say it, a professional need, whilst at the same time I feel and know that you will.'

Jim smiled. 'I'm glad you put it like that. Yes, I appreciate your supervisory concern and your personal belief in what I am doing.' He was nodding his head. 'Yes, that feels good, and, yes, I am aware that this is powerful stuff and, well, you'll be hearing more about it, that's for sure.'

'Yes. Didn't Rogers write of people as process persons, or something like that?'

'I'm not sure, but it sounds like something he might have said, or written.'

'Well, Pauline's in process – and so are you – and they are running parallel and have a point of contact once a week in which you, whilst mindful of your process, maintain an attending focus on her process. Trust it, I'm sure you will. She may take a long time on her decision, it may happen fast. But we have to be sure that it is hers and that she is clear in herself about it.'

David knew he was speaking from his own sense of how people could make a decision not thought through, or out of the reaction to a part of themselves that was not their whole person and which left them feeling – eventually – dissatisfied with the decision they had taken. The more self-aware Pauline became, the greater the likelihood that decisions she made would be right for her, even though there were always likely to be parts of herself that would have some doubts. But sometimes, so long as you knew what they were and were clear about their origin, they could be accepted as relevant but not be allowed to dominate the choice.

The session moved on to another client of Jim's. He was grateful for the discussion they had had. It had opened up his thinking and his feeling about Pauline, himself, and what was happening in the therapeutic process. He often wondered at how much material could emerge from a couple of counselling sessions. The complexity of people and of relationships never ceased to amaze him. And yet, he thought to himself, we find our way through it. Yes, making mistakes, but hopefully learning from them. So much complexity, and yet ... He felt himself smiling as he drove home later, reflecting on the supervision session, and yet it is all so simple. If only we could truly understand the meaning of love – non-possessive, unconditional love.

Points for discussion

- Evaluate your sense of David's effectiveness as a person-centred supervisor.
- What issues could usefully have been explored in more depth? Why did this not occur?
- Did you feel the balance was right between describing the client and exploring the counsellor's reactions and responses?
- How do you prepare yourself for seeing clients?
- Write your own notes for this session.

CHAPTER 7

Supervising time-limited counselling for stress in a GP surgery*

Martin is a counsellor at a GP surgery where the counselling has been taking place. One of the issues explored previously in supervision has been his feelings towards time-limited work and its appropriateness. The client, Mandy, is 36 and she lives alone. She presented with symptoms of depression and low motivation associated with her work. She has a busy and demanding job but is currently signed off from work.

In previous sessions she has released pent-up feelings associated with her mother's death five years ago, the death having occurred just before she began her present job. After the first session Mandy felt more positive and began to address work issues and the choices/options that she had. She recognised her tendency to be busy which paralleled her own mother's style of working. This recognition was a shock to her and she experienced an anxiety attack in the counselling session.

In the first supervision, Anne, Martin's supervisor, encouraged him to explore his feelings and reactions to Mandy, including his recognition that she was of an age that meant she could have been his daughter. Genuine feelings of affection for Mandy emerged, indicating the capacity of the counsellor to have feelings for the client beyond therapist–counsellor or indeed father–daughter.

In a later session, and as a result of feelings associated with making changes in the present, Mandy connects with her experience as a four year old of being taken into foster care. The changes she had had to face and endure as a child had been very painful. She began to doubt whether she could continue with her present job.

In the following session Mandy acknowledged her need to make choices as an adult woman, and in her own right. She addressed issues of identity as a woman with her own power. At the second supervision session, Martin explored the

---

* Taken from *Time Limited Therapy in Primary Care: a person-centred dialogue* (2003) by Richard Bryant-Jefferies. Radcliffe Medical Press, Oxford.

impact that Mandy was having on him, particularly when she had become her four year old self during the session. Issues of why Mandy was not expressing anger whilst anger had become present for Martin were addressed. Also, the issue of how empathic a counsellor can be when they are attending to their own authenticity, and whether there is a point of transcendence in moments of deep connection in which greater authenticity and empathy become present at the same time.

Mandy then cancelled the next appointment due to illness and at the next evidences more anger, frustration and determination. She again explores the impact on her of her mother's style of working and her need to be busy and to justify herself as being good enough. She is making plans to return to work the following week and discusses the changes she wants to make to reduce her work-associated stress. Further tearful feelings towards her mother are released as she expresses gratitude towards her mother who she realises was doing her best.

The following supervision session takes place at this point, after this latest session, with Martin intending to simply update Anne on his work with Mandy.

Supervision session

Supervisor: Anne

Supervisee/Counsellor: Martin

Client: Mandy

'I haven't so much to say about Mandy today, Anne. I have only seen her for one appointment since I last saw you as she was unwell one week. Mind you, the session that we did have was a bit of a roller-coaster ride, well, it was right at the end.'

'So it got a bit, what, intense?' Anne replied, wanting to clarify a little more what it had felt like.

'Very intense. Suddenly Mandy started grieving heavily for her mother, completely out of the blue. I wasn't expecting it. The session had not been particularly emotional, but just as we were into the final ten minutes and the session seemed to be winding down, well, it took me by surprise.'

'Mhmm. Really took you by surprise.'

'Yeah. Up until then the session had largely focused on what changes she was going to make when she returned to work.'

Anne was aware of frowning slightly, she had the idea that Mandy wasn't heading back to work just yet, somehow she had got the idea that she was going to be off for a while. She voiced her thoughts. 'I was thinking Mandy was going to be off work longer. Did I get that wrong?'

'No, I was expecting her to be off work, in fact the GP had dropped in on the day that Mandy did not attend and wanted to know how she was getting on. I didn't disclose much, but we did talk about how much time she might need to get ready to return to work, and we both felt it would take a while. Anyway, the next time Mandy saw Dr Hill she had persuaded Dr Hill that she was ready to go back to work, and that was that. Mandy goes back next week, and I see her for her last session next week.' Martin was aware of his own unease coming back over all of this although he couldn't really say why. It just seemed too quick, somehow, given the depth of the conditions of worth that Mandy had experienced as a child when she was fostered out and the impact of her mother with her focus on work and being busy.

'You don't look too comfortable about it, Martin.' Anne was noticing that Martin didn't seem too relaxed, he looked a bit tense as he had been talking.

'I'm not, but I can't really be specific about it. I just sense that Mandy is hoping to have changed around a pattern that has been stuck for life in, what, five sessions. And I have my doubts. But I also have to say that I hope she has. Maybe she has made enough change in herself to sustain a fresh approach to working and her lifestyle generally. I really hope that she has if that is what she wants. But I know I'm not sure.'

Anne nodded. She was thinking about how a limited period of counselling could leave counsellors feeling that the work had only really just begun. It could mean a sense of incompleteness and lack of a sense of fulfillment in the counselling process. Yet forced closure on the counselling relationship did not mean that the client stopped working on the issues. The client's growth process would continue and often the hard part for a counsellor lay in accepting that they would only travel part of the journey with their client, and that they had to let go and trust that they had helped the client become more self-aware and able to choose, or develop, a way of being that satisfied them. 'So, not sure whether the changes she is planning can be sustained and built upon. To you it feels as though five sessions is too short.'

Martin sat thinking for a minute. Yes, he thought, I know what it is. He voiced his thoughts. 'It's the falseness of it all that is troubling me.'

Anne was unsure what Martin meant. 'Can you tell me more?'

'Mandy is going back now partly because she wants to try it and still have a session to talk it through with me. I don't think she would be choosing to go back if the counselling was on-going. I have a sense, and I could be wrong because I don't know what Mandy is thinking or feeling about this, it is an assumption. But I think that Mandy is wanting to use our last session as a kind of safety net because she isn't sure either. I'm sure she wants to feel she will be able to come back and say how well she has done and to be able to end the counselling on a really positive and encouraging note. But there is a risk of it not being quite like that, and maybe part of her recognises this and also sees that final session as a support if things go wrong, or don't work out as she is planning.'

'I'm struck by a sense of she hasn't a lot of time at work any way, what, three days before she sees you? Not much time to really know how she is coping and making changes.'

'Yeah. But I am still aware that these are our thoughts, and I don't know what is motivating Mandy to go back now, other than she did emphasise the idea of going back and having that final session afterwards. That seemed to be coming across to me as the main reason. She talked of having more energy but ..., I don't know. I'm concerned. I felt that in the session but didn't voice it. I really didn't want to undermine her. She could be right. She may have done enough, but I know I'm not convinced.'

Anne was reflecting on whether to hold Martin with his concerns and allow him to explore them, or shift to what he felt he needed to do about his concern. She chose the former, that being where Martin actually was in himself at this time. 'Is she going back too soon and has the fact of there being only the one session left encouraged her to return to work sooner rather than later? You don't know, you're concerned.'

'Yeah, I am. But I don't know whether to say anything.' Martin thought for a moment and realised, of course, that he couldn't plan to say anything as he didn't know what Mandy would experience in those first three days back at work. He felt he would know what to say when they met up next week, but what he could sense nagging at him now was why he hadn't said anything in the session. 'Maybe I should have said something in the session, Anne, maybe I should have trusted myself in what I was experiencing, and Mandy to hear it as a concern rather than as a questioning of her decision.'

Martin's uneasiness and lack of trust (of himself and Mandy) has obstructed his ability to be transparent. This is crucial. The ability of the person-centred therapist to be congruent plays an important part in creating the therapeutic climate within which the client can undergo constructive personality change.

'Never any guarantees how a client will hear something that you say, but your wonder now is whether you should have said something. You lost your transparency.'

'I did. I can see it now. I didn't want to undermine Mandy.' Martin thought for a moment and he began to feel he was getting some clarity about what was happening. 'You, know, it seems as though it isn't only Mandy who has adjusted to making what feels like for her the best use of the six sessions. So am I.'

'So you feel that you have both in some way adjusted to the time-frame that you have.'

'Yes. I mean, I was holding back because I wanted Mandy to leave the session with the confidence that she came with, and I didn't want to risk undermining that. Had we more sessions not just one more, I think I would have said something, in fact, I'm sure I would. But it is as though it became harder for me to be congruent because I was thinking this way.'

'Makes short-term work quite challenging to our approach where the counsellor's ability to be congruent is such an important element in the therapeutic work.'

'Yes.' Martin replied, 'it does, but that is no excuse. However long I have with a client, I need to bring my authentic self into that therapeutic space. I haven't been as helpful to Mandy as I could have been.' Martin reflected for a moment and he was aware of feeling somewhat pissed off with himself. He continued, 'makes me feel somewhat pissed off with myself, yet it feels like the moment has passed now. Whether I say anything next session will depend on what transpires in the session. But there were things I could have said last session, I'm sure.'

'So your sense is that you weren't helpful to Mandy but that the moment may have passed. What might you have said?' Anne was feeling that it could be helpful for Martin to bring into words whatever was on his mind, if only to release it.

Martin thought back to the session. How had it gone? What had Mandy being saying, and what had he been feeling? 'I remember my unease when Mandy said she was going back. I said something like, "so, going back next week then", and I remember trying to say it in a kind of bland sort of way, not wanting it to sound doubting of the wisdom of it, and yet not sounding totally devoid of feeling. It felt wrong somehow, I just wasn't expressing what I was feeling and thinking. It wasn't a congruent response. It was incongruent. But I justified it to myself by deciding to maintain my empathy on Mandy. But . . . I don't think I made the right choice, Anne. It troubles me.'

'Troubled by your incongruence in that moment', Anne replied seeking to hold the focus on Martin's discomfort.

'I didn't want to cause her to feel I didn't support her in her decision.'

'Mhmm.' Anne could feel herself wanting to know why, wanting to clarify what this was about. 'I feel I really want to ask "why?".'

Martin sighed, 'I don't know. I could have said something like, "You're really sure it is time to go back?" but even then I can feel myself thinking, yes, but I'd have to say it in a way that won't upset her or direct her away from her own decision.'

'Not directing her away is an appropriate reason, but not upsetting her?' Anne was aware of feeling concerned.

Clients have a right to feel how they need to feel. Martin would not be deliberately seeking to cause upset, he would be being transparent as to his genuine concerns. How the client then reacts is according to their needs. What has happened is that Mandy has effectively been directed away from the opportunity to explore whatever might be present for her if she engaged with the thought that she could be going back too soon.

'I think I'm struggling a bit with theory here. I mean, I don't want to be directive and I don't want to question her own internal process of evaluating her situation and formulating a response that is realistic to her. God, that sounds a mouthful. But I want to feel able to be authentically me, and I wasn't.' Martin sat back in his chair. 'I got pushed out of my congruence, Anne, I can see that. I got blocked, and I know the block was coming from me. I don't believe that the client made me behave this way. I made a choice, and I am damn sure it wasn't the right one, or let's say the most therapeutically helpful one. Dammit, I'm supposed to be authentic with my clients, I owe them that at the very least.'

Anne had noticed that Martin had raised his voice and looked more than a little heated. 'You sound pretty fired up about all this, Martin.'

Martin felt the smile spontaneously spread across his face. 'You know, I said something about being fired up to Mandy in that session. What was it? Yeah, she'd been talking about going back to work and her drive to be busy, and then said something about having a bit of energy and immediately feeling she had to go back to work. That's right, she had begun to question herself about going back to work. Oh, yes, and there had been a discussion around whether her drive to be busy was learned from her mother or something more genetic and deep-seated, and did that mean she was powerless to change. Anyway, she got very fired up, angry, not wanting to make the same mistake of overdoing it, wanting to be in control. I remember she said she was quite angry with herself.'

'Angry with herself.'

'And frustrated as well. She went on to talk about feeling like she had got into this damn rut, and that she had to get out of it and learn to stay out of it. She was very determined and I remember matching her tone of voice. Then she suddenly went quieter, having got a sense of the immensity of the changes before her. But then she got back into that stronger part and affirmed how she had to change, that she had to move on and make choices that kept her away from that busy, busy, busy pattern.'

'You know, there's a word that I haven't heard you use but it is very present for me as I hear you speaking, Martin. *Desperation*. It all sounds very desperate.'

'Yes.' Martin thought for a moment, yes, that really did sum it up, and he suddenly became aware of the tension in his own body. He had sat forward again in his chair and his back had tightened up. He sat back again. 'It's leaving me with a lot of tension, I know that.'

Anne decided to stay with this although she was still carrying concern from earlier linked to how Martin, whilst saying he was non-directive, had unwittingly directed Mandy away from focusing on the concerns that were present about her going back too soon. But for now she wanted to stay with Martin whose body seemed to be telling him something that he needed to pay attention to insofar as his own process was concerned. 'You're feeling physically tense.'

'I am, right across my back and shoulders.'

'What does it feel like?'

'Like a heavy weight making the top of my shoulders sore, but also my back, just below the area beneath my shoulder blades.' He raised his shoulders and bent forward a little, trying to ease the knot that was present in his back. He twisted one shoulder up, then the other. 'Gee, it's tight.'

'Given how you are experiencing this tightness, Martin, can you imagine what would cause it in real life?'

'What do you mean?'

'Well, what might you have to be doing, physically, to get the sensation of tension and tightness you are experiencing?'

Martin thought about it. 'Certainly some kind of weight across the shoulders, but not just that. Maybe if I was pushing something as well. Yes, that's it. If I was pushing something. But no, my arms aren't tense. It's in my shoulders and back.' He thought about this more and tried to imagine what posture he would need to be in to experience this tightness. 'Got it! You know those images you see of oxen pulling a plough, or something like that, with the harness thing round their necks and over their shoulders. That's it. Beast of burden. It feels like a heavy weight I'm dragging behind me, but I'm doing it by pushing with my shoulders. What's that all about?' Martin stretched and yawned, trying to ease the tightness a little.

'Tired of it?', Anne responded quickly to the yawn.

'Yeah. I want to get out of it and feel free.'

'You want to feel free.'

'Yes, I sure do. God, yes.'

Anne was aware of Mandy again. 'OK, so what meaning does it have in relation to Mandy, and your relationship with her?'

'I guess Mandy must feel as though she has realised for the first time in her life that she is dragging this weight around, the way of being that she learned earlier in her life, and has now tasted something of what it is like to be free of it, or at least to have a little less weight. And I guess she wants more of that freedom. Must be a very powerful experience. You know, the thought has just struck me that I wasn't aware of feeling so stiff until I suddenly became aware of it. I know that sounds daft, but that's how it is, isn't it? We aren't aware of things until suddenly we are. Mandy wasn't aware of how she has been in terms of having learned it from her mother until she suddenly recognised it.' Martin stopped and thought for a moment. 'But how on earth did it all get into my body?'

'Good question. How on earth did it get into your body?'

Martin thought about it. He could see two possibilities. 'Well, either I have something that I feel the same way about and it has triggered that off for me in some way, making me more aware of feeling burdened, or by focusing on what is happening for Mandy something about her has got into me. But then, I don't think anything can affect me like this unless there was already something there for it to hook into or resonate with in some way.'

'OK, so you suspect there is something in you that feels burdensome, which in some way may, or may not, have a connection with what Mandy is experiencing.' Anne had an idea as to what it might be but she wanted Martin to make his own connection. She might be wrong anyway, but she kind of felt that she was right, that it was to do with the burden of working in a contained six-session way. She asked a direct question. 'What do you find burdensome, or constraining?' She added 'constraining' as it just sounded right to say it somehow.

'I don't know about burdensome but constraining immediately brings to mind this whole question of working to six sessions.' Martin stopped and an image came to mind. He smiled.

'Yes', Anne replied, 'something's made you smile.'

'Yes, well I could see myself as the oxen and what I am pushing against is the six-session limit. I'm not dragging anything, I'm pushing it with my shoulders but I'm also strapped to it.' He sighed and felt himself relax a little. 'That's it, isn't it? It's me and the limitation of six sessions, and wanting to push that boundary but I can't. And of course it is having an impact on Mandy, and I guess it has heightened in me that sense of the weight of it all. OK, I need to reflect on this some more. I need to make my peace with this time-limited way of working. I need to change my attitude. Well, maybe I need to understand my attitude more.' Martin looked at the clock.

'So, you sense a need for greater understanding of your attitude towards this way of working. Is there anything else you want to explore on this theme, Martin?'

'No. I've spent much more time than I planned talking about Mandy, but it has been really useful. And it has certainly given me something to think about. I haven't been owning my true feelings about working this way, have I? I mean, I knew I wasn't at ease with it, but it runs deeper than that. I need to think more about it and reflect on whether there are other aspects to me that feed into it. Seems like it could be an issue to explore in personal therapy, or in the group of counsellors that I meet up with who also work in Primary Healthcare. I think I'll start with the group, we meet up again in two weeks, and I'll raise the issue there. See what happens. And I my take it to therapy, and I may bring it back here as well.'

At what point does an issue become a factor for personal therapy rather than supervision? I do not believe in rigidity regarding this. There is surely something of an overlap. Where a reaction from a counsellor can be dealt with in supervision without it impacting on the need to spend time on other work, then that seems appropriate. However, where an issue comes up again and again, then clearly it has not been resolved and personal therapy is the place to take this.

Person-centred supervision is likely to place a lot of emphasis on the supervisee's experience of working with their clients, and the nature of the therapeutic relationships that they are building. The focus will be not so much on what is 'done' with a client, but on how the supervisee 'is' with their clients when they are involved in the therapeutic process. However, there will also be content and reaction that is clearly rooted in a supervisee's struggle to maintain congruence, empathy or unconditional positive regard due to the presence of incongruence within their own self-structure. Where this cannot be resolved in supervision then personal therapy will be required.

'Seems like you want to get to the bottom of it and yes, maybe you need some time to reflect on it, discuss it with others, but bring it back here as well because clearly it could be having an impact on your work with other clients.' Anne was aware that she hadn't forgotten about the issue of why Martin had not been authentic towards Mandy when she was talking of going back to work. 'We're still left with the issue of why you didn't voice your unease to Mandy, though.'

'Yes, I'd forgotten that. You're good at holding on to issues and bringing them back. OK. I need to think about this a moment and get back into that focus.' A thought struck him almost immediately. 'I think I have a sense of what it was, and talking about what we have just been addressing I think has loosened it up for me. I think it is something to do with wanting to feel that Mandy has moved on within the six sessions, and not wanting to say anything that would undermine that. I think the six-session limit is encouraging me to want my clients to reach their goal, and maybe it is this that blocked me from voicing my unease. Maybe I didn't want her to start doubting what she had planned to do. I wanted to keep her process nicely fitting within the six-session box. Does that make sense? It does to me, and that's scary because it is changing how I work. And I'm not sure about that.'

'So you think that the boundary of six sessions affected whether you were able to be authentic with your client, fearing that she might not do as well, or at least leave the final session with unmet needs?'

'Yes, and I know that it is ridiculous in a sense. I have to trust the client's own process and their recognition that they have six sessions and that is the time-scale that they work to. And I can see that Mandy is doing this as well in terms of her timing to go back to work. Seems like she has adjusted to it and I'm struggling with it. I've got to get clarity on this, Anne, and think about my own practice in this context. I know that I can apply a person-centred approach to any time period. Wasn't Carl Rogers asked once what he would do if he had only ten minutes with a client and he replied he would offer them ten minutes of therapy!' Martin was not best pleased with himself as he really had a clear sense that he had not adjusted to six-session working and that he needed to resolve it. But at least it did help him make sense of his lack of authenticity.

'Yes, we have to work within the limits of what is available, and so long as it is clear and visible to the client then we must trust that they will use that time in whatever way their own actualising tendency urges them. And yes, there will be times when it will not be enough and we have to then refer on.'

'Yes. I guess I'm accustomed to working with people through a whole therapeutic process and I get frustrated if I feel I can only go part of the distance because of external factors that I have no control over.' Martin looked at the time. 'I really do need to spend a little time on other clients Anne. I will give more thought to all of this, but I would like to move on.'

'I hear you say you want to move on, but there is still something nagging at me and I need to bring us back to it. You mentioned earlier that mentioning your concerns would have to be done in a way that won't upset her or direct her away from her own decision. "Won't upset her" does not feel comfortable. We are not there to direct or protect clients from their discomfort, you know that, so what was that about?'

Martin smiled, 'I love the way that you remain open to your feelings and express them. It's exactly what I was struggling with.'

'I was aware that it might be tempting not to say anything as we had moved on, but it remained present, and I was aware of the risk of parallel processing.' Anne was aware that she didn't want the focus to slide back to theory. Anne decided to make the focus clear and sharp. 'So, you didn't want to upset Mandy.'

An example of parallel processing is where some pattern of behaviour in the counsellor–client relationship gets lived out in the supervisor–supervisee relationship. In this case, Martin's inability to voice his authentic concerns and be transparent to his client could have been paralleled by Anne not mentioning her concerns regarding Martin saying he didn't want to upset his client. These kind of dynamics have to be watched for. The supervisor's heightened self-awareness and congruence provides the means whereby he or she can sense whether she is acting out of character. Sometimes it goes unnoticed in the session but the supervisor may then carry this process into their supervision and it is hoped that it will be recognised then.

'No, I didn't, but I'm really not sure why. Was I protecting her? Was I wanting her to succeed and felt I might ...' Martin had a sudden thought. 'I'm wondering whether I felt she had had enough upset over those sessions. But that's ridiculous. I know that isn't how I feel about this work, but there is something about Mandy, isn't there? But I don't know what it is. Of course I can't go around stopping my clients getting upset. That really is a personal therapy issue, Anne. My sense is that this is only a Mandy-oriented reaction on my part, but I need to talk this through and get into my own experiencing on this. I think that my now heightened awareness of it is going to help me offset it if it comes up again in our final session. But I do want to get to grips with this and if there is a block in me then I have to find out what it is and explore it. I do think it is linked to my work with Mandy, though.' Martin sat and ran images of his other clients in front of him, trying to discern whether he sensed he had in any way been blocking them from being upset. It just didn't ring true as he thought of recent sessions with these clients. 'I'm just thinking about my other clients, but I can't see anything to indicate I'm not letting them get upset. If anything, it feels the opposite! Personal therapy and I'll also keep you informed of what I get from it, Anne. Do you think that's the best way forward?'

Anne felt at ease with this. The tension she had been carrying around this issue had lifted. She was glad she had voiced it and that Martin had responded positively. He could have been defensive, but one strength of Martin's that she admired was his commitment to his on-going personal development so that he could be fully and authentically present within the therapeutic relationship. 'That feels OK, Martin, and I'd be interested to know what you find out as it would be useful for me to be mindful of in future supervision sessions.'

'No problem, I can appreciate that. So, shall we move on?'

After the supervision session, and on his journey home, Martin was thinking about how he really needed to trust Mandy's own actualising tendency, that she was making choices that, given the context, were most reasonable and which, for her minimised the risk of anxiety and discomfort. Yes, there was a lot of hurt associated with her past, and it had left her with particular personality traits that she now had mixed feelings about. Yet she was an adult and capable of making her own decisions. As he pondered on this Martin was aware that he was beginning to feel somehow uneasy about something. What had triggered it off? He pulled the car over into a lay-by. He just sensed that something important was moving around on the edge of his awareness, but he couldn't quite grab hold of it.

The words that started to come back to him more forcibly were those he had just been thinking about, 'she was an adult and capable of making her own decisions'. Of course he knew that. She was a successful career woman, making decisions and choices all the time and, OK, so she had become overwhelmed, but she was certainly capable of making decisions. He recognised that the therapeutic process of counselling had helped her to re-think her attitude towards work and to plan changes. Yet he was still uneasy.

As he was sitting there trying to make sense of it he realised that in fact his mind had begun to go blank, he was just sitting, staring out of the window but without really taking anything in. Suddenly the words from that earlier session came forcibly to mind. He heard Mandy saying them, 'please don't make me'. He felt the goosebumps break out over his arms and up his neck. And he felt tears in his eyes and a lump in his throat. He closed his eyes, trying to stay with the feelings that were beginning to clarify inside himself. Fear. Fear of the unknown. Loneliness. The sense of not being heard. Abandonment. Powerlessness. All the feelings that a four year old might experience when made to do something she did not want to do, or lose something that was precious and familiar. The feelings began to subside and Martin took a deep breath and blinked, seeking to bring himself back to focus yet also wanting to honour the presence of what he was feeling.

My God, he thought, I'm still carrying that and it is very much present. He then began to wonder what effect it may have been having on his work with Mandy. It suddenly came to him that he had not really been fully relating to her as an adult. He couldn't have been with this strength of feeling present towards her as a little girl. Had he been trying to protect her in some way? Oh-oh, he was filled with a disturbing thought. She's just about young enough to have been my daughter. Was I wanting to offer her more sessions because I wanted to protect her and support her? Was I allowing a kind of fathering impulse to get into the sessions? He was aware that he was now very much back in his head, trying to think back. Had that been why he had felt so uneasy at not voicing his concern? Was it more than feeling time was limited?

He continued to reflect on this insight and didn't reach any firm conclusion. But he acknowledged to himself that he needed to be aware that perhaps he was not fully engaging in an adult to adult relationship in the counselling, or at least, he was at risk of slipping away from it. He asked himself whether he really thought of Mandy the adult as a daughter figure, and the more he thought about it, the more that didn't feel how it was. No, it was her as the four year old that was making the impact, but could that still have affected him when he was with her and when she was not expressing that aspect of herself?

He made a mental note to take that back to supervision. But he knew he wanted to clear this in personal therapy. It had hooked into him and that meant there was something within himself that was sensitive to this area of experiencing. He did not believe feelings were transferred into him for no reason, but rather that they had a powerful impact because there was something about himself that resonated to the feeling tone of the client. He had to look at himself. If he had sensitivities that he was not aware of but which were affecting his behaviour, then he was being incongruent. And that was not good enough. He was aware that Mandy only had one more session, but she might come back for more and he needed to develop clarity as to the true origin and nature of his feelings. OK, time to head off. He sat up a little more upright in the seat, turned the key in the ignition and turned back on to the road.

Clients can and do have a powerful impact on counsellors and sometimes the full impact is not recognised at the time, but can make an impression later. Martin clearly needs to work this through. It is OK to be affected by clients, in fact, some would argue it is necessary to be an effective therapist. But the counsellor needs to be aware that he or she is affected and how. Otherwise, congruence is lost and behaviours within the therapeutic setting may emerge that are at the very least unhelpful and at worse damaging to the client. Martin may be advised to at least discuss this with Anne on the 'phone before he sees Mandy again.

Points for discussion

- If you had been Anne, would you have responded to Martin differently, and if so, how?
- Discuss what kind of issues you might be particularly sensitive to and are at risk of being incongruent around.
- What issues do you experience in yourself regarding working in a time-limited way?
- Critically evaluate Anne's work in this session. Do you feel the issues that needed to be addressed were addressed as fully as necessary?
- Is this a situation in which Martin should talk through with Anne his experience in the lay-by before he next sees Mandy?
- Write supervision notes for this session.

CHAPTER 8

Supervising the counselling of a young man seeking to find identity and independence*

Peter is a client who has been attending counselling for just a few sessions. He is seeking to find a greater sense of his own identity as a man and to free himself from his relationship with his mother. His difficulties are rooted in experiences of rejection from an early age, yet which also left him continuing to seek the love and approval that as a child were not offered. During the course of the counselling he has recovered a memory from the past. It was connected with an experience in an earlier counselling session when his throat was dry but he felt unable to ask for a glass of water.

As a young child he had gone to his parents' bedroom in the night to ask for a glass of water and been shocked by his mother waking and telling him to get out. He re-lived the experience in a session through the following experience.

The noises stopped, abruptly. He heard movement. The light came on, the bedside light. He saw his mother, his mummy, he wasn't sure which she was – his mummy, but ... Peter was flooded with feeling and emotions. He was suddenly two people. He could feel utter confusion and shock – coming from himself, from somewhere deep, from within his smallness – and absolute horror from himself as he was looking on. He was transfixed, staring at the image before him, but was it before him, as it was in his head. He couldn't think about it, he just sat, standing, watching, frozen, horrified. Who was that man? Who was he? He didn't know him. It wasn't his daddy, his father.
'Go away. Go a-waaaay!' The voice screeched in his brain, but it wasn't in his head but outside of his head as well. His mummy, his mother, screaming at him to go away. But he couldn't go. He couldn't move. Peter the adult sat, unable to move. Peter the child stood, unable to move. Both icy cold. Both connected in time in the horror of a singular moment of experience.

---

* Taken from *Relationship Counselling: Sons and Their Mothers: a person-centred dialogue* (2004) by Richard Bryant-Jefferies. Radcliffe Medical Press, Oxford.

Peter is now 28 and continues to live at home with his mother. After his father died, some five years or so previously, he had felt he needed to be there with and for her. Both his brother and sister had previously left, each in their own way eager to get away. None of them had felt wanted. His father had not been very powerful in the parental relationship, he tended to retreat into his hobbies, and Peter has no idea who the man was that he saw in bed with his mother, but he never saw him again.

In previous sessions he had talked about his father's death and had been quite ambivalent as to whether counselling was right for him. He has described a dream related to his being at a cross-roads – well, more of a fork in the road – and of hearing his father's voice urging him on. Peter did not attend one appointment, following on from a difficult session in which he became very uncomfortable as a result of Michael drifting during the session and the interaction became quite stilted as a result. However, he later realised this was a mistake and resumed contact, partly because of feeling inspired and energised as a result of listening to Meat Loaf singing 'Bat out of Hell', which spoke to him in relation to his need to get out of his mother's home and to build his relationship with Melanie a woman from work that he has recently asked out, and with whom he seems to be getting on well with.

The following supervision session follows on from the counselling session in which the memory is recovered. Suzy is Michael's supervisor.

Supervision session

Supervisor: Suzy

Supervisee/Counsellor: Michael

Client: Peter

Client's girlfriend: Melanie

Michael had begun by describing what had been happening in his sessions with Peter. Suzy listened and noted a sense that Michael was uneasy. She couldn't quite put her finger on it, but there was something about the way he spoke that left her feeling that in some way he was not comfortable with what was happening. She noted it and waited to see if it would pass.

'So, he has reconnected with a memory from his early childhood and now he has to somehow integrate that into himself, and into his life and his relationships, particularly towards his mother.' Michael paused. 'You know, I really feel for him. It's hard to imagine quite what it must be like to recover a memory like that. I mean, I guess at some level, he knew. I mean, the memory was stored somewhere, but out of reach – at least from his waking consciousness, if I can put it like that.'

Suzy empathised with his feeling, 'yes, something about his situation really touches you'.

Michael nodded. He'd been left with a clear image of the look on Peter's face as he had re-lived that experience. It had made a profound impression. So much expression. Michael felt quiet and he simply nodded in response to Suzy.

Suzy noted the silence and it felt different, meaningful in some way. It felt important to stay therapeutically connected with Michael. She wasn't his therapist and she had no intention of drifting into that place, yet she sensed that something was happening for Michael and she knew she needed to help him. Nothing outwardly, nothing he had particularly said, but it was a sense she had – call it an intuition perhaps – and she had learned to trust such subtle promptings.

Silences are moments of communication. It may be that what is being communicated is the sense of someone not knowing what to say, but it can also mean that the person simply has nothing to say. It can also indicate that internal processes are occurring and the supervisee needs to attend to them, with the supervisor waiting until they are ready to share, if they choose, what has been occurring for them.

It is also worth noting the use of the word 'intuition'. This comes into play from a deep sense of connection. The supervisor must be authentically present and empathically responsive to the supervisee. Then the inner, subtle promptings are more likely to be trustworthy. Where these connections are not present, then any urge to speak or act is more likely to be emerging from the supervisor's own issues and is likely to cut across the supervisory process. Having said that, if the connections are not present then it is debatable as to whether supervision is actually taking place at all in any genuinely meaningful sense.

Michael looked across at Suzy. She seemed very calm, a slight smile but without smiling, seemingly inviting him to say more, to express what was present for him. He took a deep breath though his lips remained tight. After a few more moments he began to share his feelings.

'I somehow seem to be feeling quite overwhelmed by the magnitude of what Peter is facing. Here we are, talking about it, and somewhere out there Peter is doing whatever he needs to do to come to terms with what has happened.'

'Mhmm, somewhere out there. And it affects you.' Suzy kept her response minimal, and open. She waited.

'It does affect me. I mean, I know I trust his process, and all that. I know that the actualising tendency will seek a constructive expression in response to what has occurred. I know that . . .' His voice seemed to trail off.

'You know that . . .' Suzy reflected his words and his style of speaking.

Michael was shaking his head, yes he did know it, and yet . . . somehow, and he was somewhat surprised and unnerved by it, but he could feel a sense of unease, of somehow not being quite so sure. 'I do know that, and yet . . .'

'And yet ...?'

Michael was shaking his head again. 'It seems so immense.'

'Mhmm. Such an immense thing to face.'

Michael was aware that he felt quiet inside as he was speaking. Yes, he knew the actualising tendency moved people towards fuller functioning, towards a more fulfilling way of being, or at least a way of being that most effectively met the individual's perceived needs. And yet ... there was something about what Peter was facing up to, and it seemed to be touching something very deep within Michael as he sat there, reflecting on the therapeutic process.

Moments of reflection are important in supervision. Here, the supervisee is in touch with his feelings and his thoughts. Thoughts and feelings are relevant. It is a myth that counselling is simply about feelings. The therapeutic process is about engaging with the whole person. Michael has been left thinking about Peter, and Suzy lets him flow with his thoughts, trusting that his process will take him to where he needs to be, and that it will have relevance for his work with Peter.

Michael closed his eyes. 'Where do you begin, I mean, where does Peter begin? His world can never be the same. He knows something, really knows something, about his mother, about himself. He knows that his mother rejected him, refused to meet his needs, and in a highly emotional moment when, as a young child, he sees this strange man in bed with her. I mean, what did he think? Well, maybe he didn't, maybe he just felt but was unable to process the feelings.' Michael paused and thought back to the last session. 'Well, he's re-engaged with them to some degree. What it will lead to, how he will become, I don't know.'

Suzy responded to what she felt was present, 'sounds like you want to know.'

'Yes, I really wish I could see how this is going to turn out. One moment in that session he seemed determined to leave – oh yes, he talked about wanting to leave like a bat out of hell reference to some record – I don't know, not my scene. But he really seemed to have connected with that and then ...' Michael was speaking more slowly as he made a connection. 'Must have felt like hell in that bedroom, must have not known what to do, or what he wanted to do. Run? But which way?' He shook his head. 'Poor kid. Didn't deserve that, and, well, maybe the rejection started then, or maybe it had already begun. Kind of feel the latter otherwise you'd think that his mother would have been more caring towards him. But he doesn't remember that. Of course, he could be screening that out in order to maintain his primary sense as a not good enough boy, as someone only deserving of rejection.' Michael paused again. 'Guess it gets to me.'

Suzy nodded, and she felt it was important to help Michael clarify what he was experiencing. Peter was affecting him and that was OK, it was a sign of relationship between them, but she also needed to be sure that Michael was able to hear Peter, to hear what Peter wanted to communicate and for it not to get lost amongst Michael's own reactions.

'Gets to you, what he went through, how it affected him, how he is now.' Suzy sought to not only empathise with what had just been said, but draw together the threads that she was experiencing Michael communicating to her.

Michael had closed his eyes again and was aware of a sense of his own identity as a man, what that meant to him. He wasn't sure how his thoughts had wandered to this theme, but that was how it was. 'Leaves me thinking of myself and what it means for me to be a man, Suzy.'

'Mhmm, wondering what that does mean for you, and for Peter.'

The process has taken Michael back to his own experience, back to a question to ask of himself. Suzy's response could have been more focused – 'mhmm, what it means for you to be a man' said slowly would have been more empathically sensitive.

'There is something about what he has told me that sort of resonates, but I can't put a memory or an experience to it.' Michael was frowning as he struggled to make sense of his experience.

'Like there's something about you that resonates with Peter?'

Michael was shaking his head, 'no, not exactly. I'm not sure. It's not an experiential thing in the sense of feeling I've had his experience. I don't have a sense of rejection, I really don't and I've not unearthed anything in my own therapy, so I feel OK about that. And yet, there's still something that really touches me.' As he spoke he felt an upwelling of emotion. He found himself taking a deep breath and feeling suddenly fired up, angry. He wasn't sure where that had come from, but it was present for him as he looked over towards Suzy who continued to sit quietly, yet with a sense of curious interest in her expression.

'Mhmm, that something, that something ...' Suzy did not want to direct Michael towards any conclusion, or to actually help him to resolve his experience. Rather she wanted to give him time to reach his own conclusion which could involve him being given the space to connect with an aspect of himself, or something within his own experience that had relevance to the relationship he was forming with Peter.

He listened to Suzy, to the way she spoke, slowly and quietly. Yes, he thought, that something. And he could feel a bit of fire now, 'bloody woman', he heard himself say with some degree of passion. Suzy was slightly taken aback by the abruptness. She guessed her body language must have communicated this. She voiced her feeling, seeking to maintain her own transparency in the supervisory relationship. 'Where did that come from?' The moment she said it she realised she hadn't empathised but had rather been unable to stop herself from conveying surprise.

Michael shrugged, he didn't know and he didn't care much. 'I don't know. She pisses me off. Peter's a nice guy, but he didn't deserve any of this.'
'You really like him.'

The supervisor has directed Michael away from his feeling pissed off and angry with 'that bloody woman' and instead focused on her sense – and it is her sense – that Michael really likes Peter. She knows he does, but he hasn't actually said this. 'That bloody woman makes you angry, pisses you off and Peter's too nice to deserve any of this' might have left Michael with more freedom to choose which area he wanted to focus on and develop. Yet, as in any situation, the supervisee moves on to say what he wants, but the subtle directiveness has to be watched. It is a hard discipline to be non-directive. This disciplined aspect of person-centred working is often overlooked, particularly by other traditions and those who actually find the discipline too hard and prefer a looser approach. In fact, person-centred practice is not loose, far from it, it is disciplined and has to be in line with a set of values and principles that lie at its theoretical heart – the necessary and sufficient conditions, the power of non-directivity, and the presence and working out of the actualising tendency.

'I do.' Another pause. 'I'd hate to have to face up to what he is going through. I mean, how does it affect you? I know, you know, theoretically, and I've seen and experienced how crap in childhood affects people, gets to them, messes them up. But Peter's not messed up – he's got a good job, but he's stuck at home, wanting to get away and yet desperate to feel his mother's love – and she's not giving it.' A thought struck him and he was voicing it as he was thinking it. 'Surely a boy has a right to love from his mother?'
'A right to be loved.'
'Well, yes, I was loved.'
'Mhmm, you were loved so Peter should have been loved.'
'Yes. Dammit, I know it isn't that way for many people, and I know that love is often quite conditional – you know, I'll only love you if ... but ...' Michael paused, he knew what he was about to say, but suddenly the words weren't right. He'd wanted to say that conditional love was better than no love, but he wasn't sure. Suddenly he wasn't sure. It was an idea that he'd been aware of but it was suddenly very present for him. He didn't know why; why in this particular moment it seemed to have deeper significance, but he knew the thought wasn't something he could put into words and own.
Suzy noted the hesitation and responded, '... but ...?'
'Caught myself, wanted to say conditional love is better than no love, and yet, well, I guess I just don't know.' He grimaced. 'Love, so much comes back to it – what is it? Why the hell is it so important? But it is. We need it, like oxygen, the child crying for attention I guess in the moment that someone

responds feels different, is somehow reassured, able to feel in some way that he or she is deserving of attention. It's so difficult. So much goes on before we even have the words to describe it. How can we really understand what the child actually experiences? It must be so isolated, suddenly alone in the world having had nine months in the womb – warm, nourished, floating.' Michael was aware that he was talking a lot but he also knew it was something he felt passionate about, particularly after witnessing the birth of his own children. And, of course, somewhere deep inside himself, within his own memory lay the experience of his own time in the womb, his own birth and sudden entrance into a world no longer warm and protective, a world in which you now had to attract attention to get needs met.

'Huge contrast, and the sense of isolation strikes you.'

Michael was nodding. 'Yes, I mean, suddenly you're on your own and yet, have you really got a sense of self? I mean, at what age does the child really begin to be able to own the sense of separation. It happens the moment the umbilical cord is cut – and I often wonder whether that occurs too soon, whether it should be left intact during those first – I don't know how long – minutes held by the mother.' Michael paused again. 'Oh, I don't know, there's no doubt some good medical reason, but I just wonder if it might somehow ease the transition in some way.'

Suzy was very struck by the idea but did not know whether there were medical grounds for cutting the cord sooner rather than later.

Michael continued, bringing his thoughts back to Peter. 'I mean, was he wanted from the start? Or was he only rejected at the time of the incident when he was a child, and it continued from then?' Michael shook his head. 'I really hope he felt love when he was born.' There were tears in Michael's eyes, it had really got to him. Something about the idea of being born, of the isolation, and maybe of not experiencing that mysterious something called love. His heart went out to Peter, and he suddenly felt anger again towards his mother.

Suzy noticed the expression change on Peter's face – from sadness to a really heavy frown and a suddenly tightened jaw. 'The sadness looks like it has been replaced by anger?'

Michael is being allowed to move between his feelings, in a sense joining up in consciousness – like joining the dots to make a picture – the parts of himself that make up the person that he is. In this way he can become more fully present and there is greater opportunity for a fuller reaction to his work with his client to be made visible to the supervisor.

Michael's response that follows, however, may indicate that Suzy could have been more empathic to Michael's need to process his thoughts and feelings. Commenting on his change of facial expression has abruptly stopped his process. Such comments have their place, but a judgement and a sensitivity is involved in ensuring their appropriateness.

'Mhmm?' Michael looked up, he had been in his own thoughts – well, in truth, in his own feeling. 'Yeah, well, just thinking of his mother.' He took a deep breath.

'You feel anger towards her?' Suzy was aware that she wasn't empathising with what Michael was saying, but tending more towards speculating, and yet she was also saying nothing that hadn't been conveyed by Michael through the combination of his words and facial expression.

'Yes, I do.' He tightened his lips once more as he thought about what he was thinking and feeling. 'I have to be honest with myself, these feelings are there, and, well, I guess they may get in the way.'

'In the way?' Suzy was inviting Michael to say more about his experience.

'Of my being open, well, maybe more transparent, towards Peter.'

'So your feelings towards his mother stop you being transparent?'

'Well, I mean, they are feelings that if I was to be transparent I'd have to express.'

'Mhmm.' Suzy didn't say any more, allowing what Michael had said to stay with him. She sat and waited. Her thoughts were along the lines of, 'so, you feel these things, why hide them away?'

'I guess for me it is a question of whether I should be venting anger here and therefore being free of it when I am with Peter, or should I simply understand my anger from my process here and be open to the possibility of revealing it to Peter?'

Suzy found herself nodding. She felt that Michael had really summed up the dilemma well, and yet she was also aware of her own instinctive reaction which she voiced 'why not both, vent it, understand it and be open to expressing it with Peter?'

'I don't want to collude with his view.'

'You don't want to collude with his view of his mother?'

'Yes.' Michael knew that this wasn't right. 'But I wouldn't be colluding, I mean, I'd be owning my stuff, wouldn't I?'

'You would. So long as you say it in a way that conveys it.'

Michael nodded. 'Yes, I can't start saying stuff about her, but maybe I can be open to what I feel.' He frowned. 'And I know that, I know that I have to be open to my feelings, and yet there is something about this situation that is leaving me reluctant or unsure. And I need to understand why.'

'Unsure about being transparent, something about your relationship with Peter, or his relationship with his mother, or . . .' she didn't get a chance to continue, Michael continued for her.

'. . . or more likely my relationship with myself.'

'Mhmm, something about your relationship to yourself.' Suzy was puzzled, unsure quite what Michael was getting at. She must have conveyed that in her facial expression.

'You look puzzled.'

'I am. I'm not sure what you mean by relationship with yourself in a person-centred context, and I don't want to now go and direct us into a theoretical discussion, I'd rather stay with what it is that you experience when you say "relationship with yourself".'

> Suzy expresses her lack of understanding, and in a way that leaves Michael able to choose whether he wants to clarify what he means, or not. He has picked up on her facial expression and it is important that she is open and transparent. It actually offers Michael an opportunity to clarify his meaning further which can help him connect more accurately with his own process.

Michael paused but only briefly. 'It's like how I react to my own reactions. It's like I feel what I feel for Peter, for his mother. They are present within me and yet, well, they're not me. I mean, it's like the feelings are present and I am experiencing them, but I am somehow not them.'

'So you're not your feelings, but you have feelings?'

'That's right, and there is something about Peter and his mother – and you know, I realise I don't know her name, and part of me is curious and another part of me doesn't want to know! But there is something about ...' Michael looked down as he thought about what it was he was trying to say. It seemed difficult to put into words, and yet important. He was aware of anxiety within himself. 'It's making me feel anxious, I'm not sure why.'

'Mhmm, something about that relationship and it leaves you feeling anxious ...'

Michael couldn't grasp what it was that was present for him. It seemed like it was out of reach, on the edge of his awareness in some way. Present and yet somehow – he was going to think distant, but it wasn't distant. It was close, and he was struck by the sense that maybe it was too close. 'There's a something and I can't get hold of it, but I sense that it is getting hold of me.'

'So something, linked to their relationship, leaving you anxious, hard to get hold of and yet it has in some way got hold of you.' Suzy was really trying to get hold of what Michael was experiencing and communicating. It wasn't simply reflection she had offered, she was experiencing greater depth than the simple mirroring of Michael's words. To her they were both on a journey, feeling their way forward towards ...? She sat, seeking to remain open to what was present within her as she also maintained her focus on Michael and what he was trying to connect with.

Michael sat, tight-lipped again. He couldn't find it, connect with it. He was shaking his head. He opened up his hands almost as though he was trying to physically get hold of something, but he couldn't. He had tensed them along with his fingers, as though he was holding some large invisible ball in front of his chest. 'I can't get hold of it.'

A thought struck Suzy and she felt a strong urge to say something that wasn't directly linked to what Michael was saying, and yet .... She trusted this instinct. 'Pre-verbal?'

Michael nodded. 'Maybe. If so, then, it may mean something happened earlier that affected Peter and it's locked up in his pre-verbal experiencing and it's leaving it so difficult for us to get hold of with our adult, word-based thinking and feeling.'

> Where there is a genuine struggle to find words in supervision when discussing a client where it is known that significant and damaging events occurred early in life, it can be – though it does not have to be – an indicator of something having happened when the client was at a pre-verbal age. The experience has been symbolised without the use of language, a cluster of feelings and sensations that may later re-emerge – powerfully but without a clear vocabulary to describe what is present and what occurred.

They both sat for a while in silence, each contemplating what had been said, and the implication. Of course, neither knew the reality, in many respects it was speculation, and yet . . . Suzy had felt a strong sense of the idea that the struggle was to put something into words that was perhaps contained within Peter's experience in a form that wasn't word-based. And she also believed that everyone had that place in themselves, for everyone had a pre-verbal phase of existence where experiences were processed in a very different way.

Michael was aware of feeling rather detached, of sitting as a kind of observer of himself and the dialogue he was having with Suzy. He voiced his experience. 'It's leaving me feeling rather detached – watching myself and our conversation.' He paused to scratch his left shoulder which was itching. He even felt detached from the itch as well. It wasn't a feeling he had when he had arrived earlier, it had rather developed during the session, but more particularly these last ten minutes or so. And he was aware that the supervision session was nearly over.

'Like you're detached from what's happening?'

'Observing. Like I'm not really feeling.' He snorted. 'What was I saying earlier about not showing my feelings about Peter's mother? Now I don't seem to be in touch with feelings at all!'

Suzy responded, 'like you're cut off from feelings. They're there but you're not experiencing them, or they're just not there?'

'I'm sure they're there but I'm back from them in some way. Funny, I'm still thinking back to what we discussed earlier. Not showing feelings and then, now can't.'

'I'm wondering what was the process we went through – you went through – to reach this place and what significance that journey had, what were the main features?'

'Having feelings and not being them. Being uncertain, no, anxious, about transparency. Almost like I approached the idea of being transparent but then, well, here I am being anything but transparent.'

'You're being as you are. We don't understand what is happening, but you are being as you are, as you need to be, and it seems to me you are bringing it into our relationship and communicating it. It's just so very difficult to communicate and there is this sense of being detached within yourself, if that is the right way of expressing it. And there is the pre-verbal idea we touched on as well. It's all very powerful stuff. And I sense you as being present, but in the midst of, I don't know, a . . . a . . . , well, a something.'

'Yes, it's like a something that I can't put into words. There's something about Peter not being able to connect with something. That word keeps coming up now. But that's how it is. He's connected to an experience in childhood – a really painful and difficult, and wholly rejecting experience. He wouldn't have been able to make rational sense of it, but maybe blamed himself in some way. That's speculation. But anyway. And maybe behind it all is something else. And that's also speculation.'

'Yes, lots of speculation all of a sudden. We don't know. We really don't know, and perhaps we have to accept that and be open to that not knowing. It's OK not to know.'

A broad grin broke out on Michael's face, and he could suddenly feel some kind of change taking place inside himself. It was clearing, he was feeling clearer. It was like a fog had lifted. Yes, he thought, yes. He was smiling even more as Suzy asked him what had happened.

'Maybe for us, but for Peter, he's got to know something, he's got to know that he's loved. He's got to feel that love. He's got to have that affirmation that in the eyes of his mother he is lovable. Back to needing love like oxygen. He knows he needs it, but that need, that urge is being driven from his pre-verbal development.' Michael was feeling clearer still as he developed his train of thought and continued to speak. 'He's got to know. He can't allow himself to doubt it. He's got to know. He's got to feel love – and I imagine as well there is a part of him in utter fear of opening himself to the possibility for fear of rejection once again.' He felt the goosebumps breaking out on his back and neck, and somehow for Michael there was a very clear knowing that what he was saying did reflect Peter's experience. And he felt so different, so much lighter.

'You look more alert, more present somehow, more sort of animated.' Suzy had been struck by a change, 'and it feels like there's more connection as well.'

Michael nodded. 'I feel lighter. Something's cleared, shifted. It seems like I needed time wallowing in it before I could emerge from it.'

'I'm aware that we don't have much time left, but I want to say that it may have needed time. Perhaps the experience you have had represents something happening for you that is either about processing your reaction to Peter and his mother, or it is something that may leave you relating to him from a different place within yourself. Maybe?' Michael took a deep breath, and then paused. He cocked his head slightly to one side as he looked over to Suzy. 'You know, it's like I have cleared something but I couldn't tell you for the life of me what it was. But something has happened. Something has changed. It's like . . . it's the pre-verbal again. I can't put it into words, but there's a shift and there is clarity and lightness. Maybe I'd simply picked up on stuff that I needed to put down, let go of, process – what do we mean by these words?'

'Maybe you have needed to be as you have been this session and, well, we do not know the reason and we do not know the result. We must trust that what has happened has value, even if we cannot explain it.'

The session closed with Michael feeling a strong sense of motivation towards his work with Peter, and yet he noted, as he thought about it on his way home, it wasn't that he wanted to make Peter different or do something. He realised he had been holding those thoughts and feelings, but now he somehow felt himself more accepting. Not a specific acceptance of one thing or another, but a general acceptance of Peter, his mother, the process they were experiencing, and the fact that he was being brought into relationship with that process. Yes, more of a motivation to be in the process. He wondered what would happen next, whether he might be different when he next saw Peter. He didn't know and, in many respects he was aware of thinking that it didn't matter. He'd be how he needed to be, and yes, yes, maybe how he needed to be would turn out to be more transparent. He smiled as he realised he was looking forward to the next session and to being in the process that was therapy.

Points for discussion

- Note down your immediate reaction to this supervision session, and reflect on how it has affected you.
- How helpful was Suzy? What in particular stands out for you from her responses to Michael?
- Is there anything that you would have responded to differently, and why?
- Were the principles of person-centred working applied to the supervision session? If not, what might have more accurately expressed a person-centred process?
- Can you think of instances in supervision where a lack of words could have indicated issues from a pre-verbal age for a client being discussed?
- Write supervision notes for this session.

CHAPTER 9

Supervising the counselling of a mother who is struggling to cope with her son's cannabis use and mental health disturbance*

Fareeda is a muslim woman who was encouraged to come to counselling by a friend. She recommended her to come to Carla, someone who the friend had also seen for counselling in the past. Fareeda has been struggling to support and cope with her elder son, Ali, who has for some years evidenced symptoms of a mental disturbance. In the counselling sessions there has already been a dialogue around ethnic and racial differences, and Carla took her reactions to William, her supervisor, in a previous supervision session.

Themes of spirituality have also been explored, with Fareeda sharing prayers with Carla, and being touched by Carla's interest and receptivity. She has also made clear her struggle to make sense of her son's condition, and her own role as his mother, in the light of her faith. She wonders what Allah is asking of her. How should she respond to her situation? She has also shared one of her son's poems in a session which summed up his desperate state of mind at a particular period in his life.

Ali recently experienced a psychotic episode, as a result of which he has been taken into hospital for treatment and stabilisation. Carla has been updating William on the situation.

---

* Taken from *Responding to a Serious Mental Health Problem: person-centred dialogues* (2005) by Richard Bryant-Jefferies. Radcliffe Publishing, Oxford.

Supervision session

Supervisor: William

Supervisee/Counsellor: Carla

Client: Fareeda

Client's son: Ali

'So, Fareeda's son had to be hospitalised. I'm wondering about your reaction to that.'

Carla nodded and spoke her thoughts. 'It sounded reasonable. Clearly, things had taken a turn for the worse. I felt for Fareeda, having to cope with what happened on her own, and I hope that things went well at the discharge meeting that she was going to attend. So how do I react? Well, whilst I am aware of feeling very concerned whether being hospitalised and being given powerful medication can have an effect that blocks the client's process, I also appreciate that for some people there is simply a need for them to be in a place of safety from which a plan of action can be formulated. Clearly, Ali was losing it. How much it was cannabis induced, how much was his own thought processes running to extreme, I don't know. But there's no doubt that Ali does experience some degree of internal pain – I'm not sure what else to call it – psychological or emotional distress?'

'I guess that for me it is about checking whether your reaction to whatever treatment Ali might receive will cloud the clarity of your empathy for whatever Fareeda might be experiencing, when you next see her.'

'Yes, and because I know that I believe, passionately, that he could benefit from some kind of therapy – maybe quite intense – to help him process whatever is happening for him, I may find it difficult to be unbiased in the next and proceeding sessions.'

William nodded, pleased that Carla could recognise this, and he asked her to clarify what she meant by her use of the word 'unbiased'.

'I might carry a negative attitude towards what Ali is offered if it isn't what I believe he should receive. And that might affect my ability to really hear Fareeda. I'm not sure. I can see how easy, if he is not offered, say, some proper therapeutic counselling – and not simply medication to control the symptoms, or keyworking sessions to only deal with controlling his thinking, and/or his cannabis use, at a very cognitive and behavioural level, well, the emotional content, the deeper, internal difficulties may get missed and any, if you like, surface changes may not get underpinned by genuine personal growth and change.'

'So your concern is about whether her son will get the kind of therapy that will go deeper into the meaning of the psychotic episode.'

'And hearing you use that label or diagnosis, I feel a reaction.' Carla didn't like these kinds of labels, they always seemed to carry a social stigma. She recognised that was as much about societal fear as anything else, but nevertheless, she knew how easy it was for people to equate psychosis with madness when for some people it was simply that they experienced themselves differently. That difference may involve taking thought and behavioural processes to extremes, but she felt that somehow there was always scope for understanding, for helping people to explore themselves and, yes, there would be times when there was a genuine chemical imbalance within the person and some form of chemical treatment was required to re-balance the system. She well appreciated that and did not have any problems with it, so long as the medication used could strategically impact on the chemical need, rather than bring with it a range of side-effects that might contribute to other areas of problematic experiencing for the client. She also accepted that medication could stabilise someone where this was the case in order to enable them to more fully engage in therapy. However, she was distrustful of deciding, too soon, that clients were incapable of engaging with someone and medication being used as a first rather than a last resort.

'What kind of reaction?'

Carla described the thoughts that she had and then continued. 'I guess the thing for me is that it is so easy for clients to be blamed or diagnosed for not being cooperative when in fact it is what they are being offered, and how they are being offered it, that is contributing to them being that way.'

William nodded. 'So, from a person-centred perspective, how would you describe your position?' He felt it would be helpful for Carla to process her reaction, her thoughts and concerns in the light of person-centred theory.

'Well, first of all, there is the fact that someone else is perhaps taking a position of authority.'

'So that authority has implications?'

'Well, once someone has been given a diagnosis then the expert on what that diagnosis means can take over. And, yes, that can be highly appropriate, but where there is uncertainty over the value or accuracy of the diagnosis, well, then there becomes the risk that the client's meaning and experience – the uniqueness of what has happened to him, or her – can get lost in the generally assumed meaning and nature of that particular diagnosis.'

'So the specificity of the client's experience gets lost in a general view of what a particular diagnosis means?'

'Yes, and I am concerned that if someone cannot relate effectively to Ali, then the specificity of his experience will not be perhaps as fully communicated and heard as it might be, and so the general understanding of treatment responses to the diagnosis will be applied without their being informed by the specificity of Ali's experience. Does that make sense, or am I making this sound unclear?'

'No, it sounds clear to me. You are concerned that if there isn't accurate communication between Ali and whoever is assigned to treat him, then he will receive treatment based on general understanding rather than what is specific to his needs, his experiences.'

'And for me it is about the vulnerability of clients with mental health problems who may need a lot of time in order to feel able to communicate the specifics of their experience, who are naturally defensive because, let's say, the underlying cause of their difficulties is some kind of trauma. He may not feel able to disclose an event or series of events for a whole host of reasons, and part of this could be some degree of mental health impairment. I know how clients can need time, and psychiatric units can be intense places. You can have a lot of disturbed people together and I know how people in those settings who are sensitive, who have been traumatised, can struggle, can withdraw. I mean, in extreme cases, they may be dissociating into some place in themselves that they learned to go into, say, in childhood, in order to cope, a place where they simply had to reinforce the view that they were a bad person. Now this gets triggered and this in turn sets off a set of behaviours that reinforce that belief, which could include non-compliance with those who are trying to help them. I'm afraid I've heard the phrase, "mad, bad, or sad" too often. People need time to trust and time to feel heard and understood. They need time for the uniqueness of their experi-ence – yes, of course it might take the same form as others' – but it is their experience, and they have their own individual meanings and interpreta-tions associated with it.' Carla sighed and shook her head. 'I guess I have strong views, but they aren't just ideas I have in isolation, I have worked with people who have mental health diagnoses, and I know what I have heard them say about their treatment. Why do people go into psychotic states? How many "voices" are simply "dissociative states" emerging, or even "configura-tions within the self" that have particularly strong identities finding a way of being heard?'

Configurations within self (Mearns and Thorne, 2000) are discreet sets of thoughts, feelings and behaviours that develop through the experience of life. They emerge in response to a range of experiences including the process of introjection and the symbolisation of experiences, as well as in response to dissonant self-experience within the person's structure of self. They can also exist in what Mearns terms as 'growthful' and 'not for growth', configura-tions, the former seemingly providing a focus for the actualising tendency, the latter those that seek to block change because of its potential for disrupt-ing the current order within the structure of self. The self, then, is seen as a constellation of configurations with the individual moving between them and living them out in response to experience in the present.

Mearns suggests that these 'parts' or 'configurations' interrelate 'like a family, with an individual variety of dynamics'. As within any 'system', change in one area will impact on the functioning of the system. He there-fore comments that 'when the interrelationship of configurations changes, it is not that we are left with something entirely new: we have the same "parts" as before, but some which may have been subservient before are stronger, others which were judged adversely are accepted, some which were in self-negating conflict have come to respect each other, and overall the parts have achieved constructive integration with the energy release which arises from such fusion' (Mearns and Thorne, 1999, pp. 147–8).

Warner (2002) writes that 'dissociated experiences ... are a great deal more personified than ordinary mood states or even "configurations" ' and that, 'dissociated process seems to arise almost exclusively as a response to early childhood trauma'. She goes on to say that these dissociated parts 'seem to emerge when trauma memories are pressing to the surface' (pp. 158–63).

'That's an interesting point. As you say, certain psychotic experiences are perhaps the effect of psychological processes that may be rooted in unrecognised trauma, or in particularly well-defined configurational states that have developed as part of the normal psychological process. It seems to require, though, that whether we are talking about a "configurational part" or a "dissociative part", in order for its presence to manifest through what gets labelled as a psychotic episode, it had to be very well defined as a discrete entity, with a strong identity within the structure of self.'

'I really think that the person-centred approach has a lot to offer in understanding these kinds of experiences. I really do. And yes, as I say, of course there are people for whom there is a need for chemical treatment – long term – to address a chemical balance, a genuinely medical condition. But I wonder just how many are being treated long term through chemical intervention for states of mind that are experientially induced and need an experiential process to resolve. I come back to my albeit simplistic belief that people damaged by unhealthy and abusive relational experiences stand the best chance of resolving them through experiencing healthy relational experiences. And I think Rogers, when he emphasised his six necessary and sufficient conditions for constructive personality change (Rogers, 1957) is saying something that should underpin all treatment. I really do.'

'That there is a fundamental quality of relationship that is necessary, but clearly not always sufficient given that there could be chemical imbalance that has an organic basis.' William was careful with his wording, aware that there was and had seemed always to have been this discussion since Rogers formulated this idea as to whether the conditions were both necessary and sufficient.

'I agree. But it is a difficult area, and, yes, the approach can and does help people with mental health problems. And, yes, medication helps and is necessary in some cases, but the need for a quality and healthy relationship with people, with those who are offering treatment, has to be important. I can't see how it cannot be. Any healthcare professional, it seems to me, needs to apply Rogers' principles – I think of them as "principles of effective human relationship" – accurate empathy, congruence, warm acceptance of the client, and all communicated and received accurately by the client because there is an established psychological contact – however minimal that might be, at least to start with.'

'And the factor of it being minimal can be particularly relevant here.'

Carla nodded. 'Yes, think of the pre-therapy work that is being done, this is an important development and application of the person-centred approach. I am thinking not only of the factor of psychological contact, but also that of the different aspects of empathy that the Pre-Therapy system defines.'

In the Pre-Therapy model, a distinction is drawn between 'empathy' as described earlier, and 'empathic contact'. In a situation in which 'the therapist does not know the client's inner frame of reference', then 'the empathy is for the client's effort at developing coherent experience and expression, perhaps a form of "concretising" the self-formative tendency during these primitive phases of therapy. Prouty goes on to suggest a second level of empathy which he defines as being for 'the concrete particularity of behavioural expression', in other words, 'not focused on the generalized essence of meaning, but on the literal expressive behaviour'. The third level of empathy which he then suggests concerns 'the increase in psychotic expression as a function of Pre-Therapy'. It is worth quoting verbatim what he has to say regarding this as it is clearly a view that many mental health professionals would find challenging. 'The client needs to get worse before she can get better. The therapist needs to be empathic to an increase in delusional and hallucinatory expression, as well as to an increase in bizarre communication (strange body language, postures, language disturbance, etc.). This means being empathic to the lived experience of the psychosis itself. This is, of course, the opposite of behavioural and chemical management' (Prouty, 2002, p. 63).

William agreed. 'OK, so I know I started this discussion, and I think it is valuable and important to make these connections in our understanding of the application of our theoretical framework. I am also becoming increasingly mindful as I sit here of Fareeda, where she is in all of this, and whether you need time to process your responses to her during our time now.' He had noted a sense of Fareeda becoming less present. It wasn't that he was not attending to Carla, or believing that the focus of their exploration was important, it was, but he felt that she was being left out of the loop, as it were, and felt a need to invite her presence back into the exploration that was taking place between Carla and himself.

'I'm feeling more and more for Fareeda. Since our last supervision session I think I have felt generally more sensitive and open to her. The issues we discussed last time I feel I have been able to put to one side, and I feel I am much more in touch with her. Her son's poem touched me deeply, he has felt more present too. And in a way this brought me more into the sessions. I think it is something about being a mother myself, perhaps we became two mothers rather than counsellor–client, to some degree. Whether that's OK or not, I'm not sure, but perhaps as I think about it now that is the nature of what occurred. This has enabled me to empathise I think more fully not just with Fareeda but with the situation that she finds herself in.'

William nodded and wanted to explore this further. 'So, the sense of your being a mother, how specifically does that help you? How might that affect you as compared to a counsellor who, say isn't a mother, or a parent even, for instance, she might have been seen by a male counsellor?'

Carla thought. 'Interesting question, that. What do I bring as a mother? Maybe there is something that makes my ...', Carla paused, 'I'm not sure how best to describe this ...'

'Well, maybe just think out loud and see what emerges.'

Carla nodded as she sought to clarify for herself what she felt in response to William's question. It was a good one, and she was aware of how it was really focusing her on exactly what she was offering, and how, in a sense, that was linked to her own identity.

'I think that it has something to do with how I can be, how I may respond. I think I can come from a place of knowing from my own experience what being a mother can be like, and yet, as we know, all experience is unique with each person taking their own meaning. So it isn't like I'm an expert on Fareeda's experience because of my own. It's not that at all. But it's like, well, maybe it affects something of the tone of what I say, maybe the part of me that if you like is associated with my mothering experience somehow reaches out to the client who has their own similar yet unique identity as a mother.' Carla paused to reflect on what she had said. Did that sound right? Was it what she wanted to say?

William reflected her words back. He didn't add his view or opinion, he simply allowed Carla to hear what she had said. 'So, the part of you that is associated with being a mother somehow reaches out to the part of the client that is their identity as a mother? That what you mean?'

The words weren't exactly her own but, yes, it was something like that. 'Yes, and I'm back thinking of configurations here. If we think of person-centred theory then yes, why shouldn't there be some kind of relationship created between parts of me and parts of my client? If we take the idea that the structure of self is made up of parts, then why shouldn't the fact that within me is present a "mother part" have significance in some way for clients who either have their own version of the same part ...?' Carla paused as another idea struck her. 'But it's more than that, isn't it, because if I work with a client, as a son or daughter their sense of self that was shaped by their experience of being mothered will perhaps be responding to the part of me that is the mother. Oh, this is complex, isn't it?'

William nodded. 'Yes, it is, and yet there is also a fundamental simplicity, and it all comes back to our congruence. Can I as a person in the counselling role be fully aware of myself to the point that I can recognise all the different parts of me and understanding my own process in response to what the client is presenting to me?'

Carla took a deep breath. 'For me that emphasises even more the challenge of working to a theory in which we use ourselves, where the therapeutic process is very much centred on the relationship, on how the counsellor and client relate to one another.'

'Mhmm, so the mother part and it will have its own associated thoughts, feelings, behaviours, yes? The mother part in you, the fact that it is present and the form it takes, will convey something to the client.'

'And it may be quite subtle, mightn't it? I mean, it might simply affect the way that I speak. I may not need to disclose whether or not I am a mother, but simply my presence as a mother, how I am because of my experience, may convey something to the client who will then take from that, well, whatever they take from it. I can't define what that will be.'

'So, yes, something is conveyed ...' William empathised with Carla and left his response in the air, being aware that whilst they had acknowledged something was conveyed, exactly what hadn't been identified.

Carla was still trying to identify the illusive something. What did she bring into her relationship with Fareeda because she was a mother? What did the mothering part of her contain? 'I don't think I've voiced this to Fareeda, I'm not sure, but I don't think so. But it seems to me that what she pulls from me, and maybe this is from the mothering part of me, is a real sense of her devotion – no, hearing myself say that I know I haven't used that word. But it is a sense that I have, and I can relate to that, of her dedication, yes, that's an important word, her dedication to her son. I think that links with my experience as well. As a mother I know I will put my child first, I know that. It's what I do.'

'So devotion, dedication, both resonate to the mother in you?'

'Very much so. I have reflected on how I would be in her situation. Not in the session, but wondered how would I be? Would I be any different if my son had similar problems? Would I see them as a problem, first of all? And I'm sure I would. I'd want to help, be there for him, help him to get the help he needs. And even if I don't say this I am sure that the mother part of me brings a certain, I don't know, I nearly said authenticity, but I don't mean that. You don't have to have been a mother to be authentic. But it brings a certain – I'm almost tempted to say solidarity but perhaps I mean something more in the way of commonality.'

'A commonality ..., of experience, you mean?'

'Something like that, a kind of commonality of ...' Carla paused. A commonality of what? 'It's something about recognising that a part of me has developed out of an experience or experiences that have some link to that which has been experienced, or is being experienced, by the client.'

That sounded clear to William. 'So, and these are my words and meaning, the commonality of an experience enables you to access that part of your own experiences that have similarities, and I am also aware of thinking that there is something about context here as well. That your own experience puts you in touch with the context of mothering, in the sense that whilst you have your version of this, and so does the client, but the generalism of mothering is a commonality even though it will probably take different forms.'

Carla was nodding. 'Yes, yes, that helps me. And this brings me to realise that it has enabled me to move beyond the differences – the ethnic context – which were present early on in our relationship.'

William smiled. 'The question remains, however, was that dealt with, or was it put aside by the emergence of the mothering commonality providing the primary point of contact between parts of yourselves?'

Time was running out in the supervision session and Carla immediately recognised that what had now emerged was important and something she needed to think about. It wasn't a perspective that she had considered before. Yes, I have an identity as a mother, as a woman, and those can become the focus for my connecting with Fareeda, but where does her experience as a Muslim come in because I don't have a sense of self that has developed within that experience?

Both Carla and William felt they had a great deal to reflect on after the session had ended. The idea that the structure of self was made up of parts had enormous implications for person-centred theory and the more they thought about it, the more significant those implications were. It left Carla more aware of her own complexity and the sense that she needed, somehow, to be aware within counselling sessions of how the many parts of her were reacting or responding to her clients. She had the image of all these non-verbal dialogues taking place, some of which became actual verbal dialogues. It left her feeling quite quiet and humbled as she pondered on the vastness of the process, the complexity and yet, as well, the fact that it was simply a matter of communication and relationship. The trick, if there was one, was to be aware of the communications that were taking place (or not taking place) and shaping the quality of the therapeutic relationship.

Points for discussion

- What are your reactions to the discussion about the person-centred approach and mental health in this supervision session?
- How does person-centred theory cater for people who experience significant and enduring mental health problems?
- How do you feel about mental health diagnoses? Do they have a part to play in person-centred counselling and psychotherapy?
- Since becoming a counsellor, what steps have you taken to enhance your awareness of diversity issues concerning cultural, racial and religious difference?
- Reflect on the value of pre-therapy. How might you apply this within your own practice?
- Which of the core conditions of empathy, congruence or unconditional positive regard felt most present in the supervision session between Carla and William?
- Write supervision notes for this session.

CHAPTER 10

Supervising the counselling of a young person in his late teens experiencing psychotic symptoms associated with cannabis use*

Charlotte is working with Ali, who is in his late teens. He is the son of Fareeda. His father is white, English and he has a younger brother, Adam. Her supervisor is Matt.

Ali has been using cannabis for some years, and has begun using the stronger 'skunk' cannabis which is more powerful than the dope, grass and marihuana of previous years. It is difficult to know whether his cannabis use caused the particular mental disturbances that he has experienced – paranoia, voices – or whether it exploited a tendency that already existed. Ali has stated many times how the cannabis helps him to settle down, but clearly it has more recently exacerbated his problems.

His father doesn't want anything to do with him, in fact he wants him out of the house. His mother is supportive but feels at times at her wits' end as she tries to keep the peace and do what is best for her son.

Ali is withdrawn in the first session, he doesn't really want to say very much. He isn't sure that he wants to come back for another session but Charlotte invites him to experience a relaxation visualisation, which he does. It makes a powerful impression on him and Ali leaves feeling good and wanting to come back for more the next week. The second session Ali does not arrive and there is no communication from him. Charlotte writes to him, hoping he is OK, acknowledging that he has probably not attended for a good reason, hoping to see him the following week and asking him to make contact if he does not expect to attend.

---

*Taken from *Responding to a Serious Mental Health Problem: person-centred dialogues* (2005) by Richard Bryant-Jefferies. Radcliffe Publishing, Oxford.

Ali came the following week and has since attended the counselling sessions inconsistently. He has also missed some keyworking sessions at the drug agency where he was referred and where he is receiving the counselling. However, the service has stayed with him, seeking to maintain contact and to offer further counselling appointments, and keyworking sessions. Ali has kept to the medication much of the time, but there have also been occasions when he's given up and gone back to the cannabis. Each time it has been a reaction to a build-up inside himself, of feeling fragmented, edgy, unable to stop thoughts running in his head. It has made him depressed as well, his mood has swung but he has not had a recurrence of the experience that he had prior to going into hospital.

As the counselling sessions have continued, albeit sporadically, the relationship with Charlotte has deepened. It has been gradual. Ali has not been consistent. At times it has seemed to Charlotte as though he presents different faces at different times, moving between them. This has been touched on but not in any great depth. When he has attended Ali has been more concerned with his present than with his past. Charlotte remains unaware of Ali's childhood which he has chosen not to talk about. She has accepted this. She realises that at the moment the most intense experiencing for Ali is what is happening for him in the present. If you like, that's where the action is. She does not know if he will wish to explore beyond that, or, indeed, whether his own inner process will require this of him, or urge material from the past into sharper awareness and, perhaps, into the content of the counselling sessions.

Desmond (Ali's keyworker at the drug agency) has sought to motivate Ali to make changes to his lifestyle and he has made some progress. Ali does get out more and he has been thinking about a job, though for now he remains signed off by his GP. He has helped out at a local charity shop and that has helped him to socialise a little.

In the seventh counselling session Ali talks more openly about his past and begins a process of recognising that there are parts to him that make up who he is, and he begins to identify them. They are more associated with particular behaviours than anything else. He plans to go away and map them out. However, this does not happen. Ali has had a difficult week, clashing with his father. In the session, an exploration of this leads to an apparent 'psychotic' episode when Ali hears voices in his head urging him to leave the session and smash something. He does not act on it and further exploration leads Ali to a deeper appreciation of that part of himself that he then calls 'jailbreak'; the part that wants to break free and get away. He draws this diagrammatically and then adds another part, 'hide away'. He finds himself getting calmer. Charlotte reflects after the session about the processes that can leave people with the kind of fragmented sense of self that Ali is experiencing.

Charlotte had discussed her work with Ali on previous occasions with her supervisor, Matt. He had experience of working in a substance misuse setting with clients who had been diagnosed with mental health problems. He understood the nature and working of statutory services. Indeed, it was his experience of working in these areas that had been a major factor in Charlotte approaching him to be her supervisor. He not only supervised her work at the drug and alcohol service, but also her other counselling work.

Charlotte has not specifically spoken yet about her work with Ali in the following supervision session, but he is on her mind. She is troubled by the process of empathising with what he communicates from within his inner world, which can seem so different to anything she has experienced.

Supervision session

Supervisor: Matt

Supervisee/Counsellor: Charlotte

Client: Ali

Charlotte had been discussing one of her other clients and the theme of feeling as though working with clients whose structure of self seems to be very fragmented emerged. Charlotte commented on the challenges of this, of being able to keep her own focus.

'Of course, once we begin to accept the notion that within the structure of self there are areas of specific identity, groupings of thoughts, feelings and behaviours along the lines of configurations within the self, then we must also accept the notion that we, as counsellors, as well as our clients, are subject to this reality. We often speak of clients in this context, but the counsellor or therapist will have their configurations although personal development work should have enabled them to identify these and have perhaps more fully integrated them if there are signs of them being unduly separated from each other.'

Charlotte nodded as she listened to Matt. She was in agreement with him. 'The problem as I see it for the counsellor is when a "part" of himself or herself gets, in effect, hooked by a "part" of the client and the counsellor is unaware that this is happening because they haven't got the necessary self-awareness to identify this process.'

Matt smiled. Yes, he knew that one as well. 'I agree. That is why I think training courses should have a large self-development focus, and I don't mean simply one-to-one therapy, in fact, I think very often the main focus should be within the training programme, through encounter, allowing these processes to be identified and used as material for the training and development process. Things get taken to a therapist that emerge from the training process and can end up becoming invisible to the trainers and the trainees' colleagues. From my experience, training as a person-centred counsellor meant a lot of personal development, and processing of experience within the training context, and that seemed to be the main focus. In fact, I was lucky, I had what I would call a person-centred training to become a person-centred counsellor, and that isn't always what happens. For me it again comes back to this notion of focusing more on how we are with our clients than what we do with them.'

The supervisor makes an interesting point. What balance should there be between theory, practice and personal development on counselling and psychotherapy training courses? With an approach that is so centred on the therapeutic relationship and the counsellor's ability to offer consistent empathy, unconditional positive regard and congruence, it is arguably even more important to have a strong focus on personal development within the training programme.

'A person-centred training puts the person of the individual therapist-to-be at the heart of the training process. This is consistent with a client-centred approach to therapy, which puts the client at the centre of the process, and with Rogers' belief that the person of the therapist is significant in the therapeutic process' (Embleton Tudor *et al.*, 2004, p. 64). Further on, the authors highlight how 'training courses from different traditions pay different levels of attention to student's personal development'(Embleton Tudor *et al.*, 2004, p. 64). Indeed, with increasingly academic syllabuses the danger is that therapy training is moving more and more into knowledge and doing, and at risk of sliding inexorably further and further away from being, from facilitating would-be counsellors into becoming the congruent person that seeks to offer unconditional positive regard and convey empathic understanding to the client, whose values are naturally and congruently expressed through their practice and their presence within the therapeutic relationship. As the same authors suggest 'a person-centred training sees that the personal development of the student *is* the training, and for this reason gives it the highest priority' (Embleton Tudor *et al.*, 2004, p. 64).

'It comes back to congruence, to the counsellor knowing themselves well enough to be fully present with their client. To know the processes within themselves and their style of working. If I'm sitting in a session, listening to a client going through an intense experience, I need to be able to feel that I am clear on why I may be reacting in a particular way – whether it is my "stuff", as it were, my own conditioned reactions to something being discussed or a particular behaviour being exhibited before me, or whether I am in some way picking up on something specific to the client's process. As if someone says something and I may feel an urge to say something in response that is not an empathic response, but is something that becomes alive within me. Is it coming from a "part" of me that is conditioned into a certain perspective and reaction to what is occurring, or is it something other that may have specific meaning to the client and which, in a sense, the client is drawing out of me?'

'Can you say a little more, or give an example?'

'Yes, well, sort of. This may not be a good example, but perhaps it is. Ali, the client who has been using cannabis and had an episode in hospital following what seemed to be some kind of psychotic disturbance? You know who I mean?'

Matt nodded. Yes, he remembered him from previous supervision sessions. He had already triggered interesting discussions between them around the whole issue of defining effective treatment responses for people so diagnosed. 'Mhmm.' He didn't say anymore, wanting to leave Charlotte to pursue her own train of thought.

'Well, last session, he . . . No, let me put it in context. We had begun looking at his nature in terms of "parts" in a previous session. And he had gone away to iden-tify the parts of himself. But there had been a problem at home that had upset him – his father can get on to him – and he had smashed a vase and, well, it had really got to him. But it also contributed to him later in the session relating to parts of himself. But anyway, what happened was he had a, well, I guess some would call it a "psychotic experience" in the last session.'

Matt frowned, unsure what Charlotte meant, and immediately experienced a sense of concern both for Charlotte and for Ali 'Were you OK with what hap-pened, and Ali?'

'Yes, yes, but what was interesting was that, well, it turned out he was sitting there with voices in his head telling him to leave, to shut up, and to go and smash something. Now, he was sitting there, and he talked a bit to himself, and I responded something like commenting on how scary it must be for him to be experiencing what was happening for him. Now, he hadn't mentioned being scared. Was my response a genuine sensing of something present for him that I was picking up on, or was it part of me feeling scared by what I sensed was happening? At the time, well, it seemed to be scary for him, and I felt that what I was saying was a kind of expression of unconditional positive regard for him, hoping to help him tell me what was happening, helping him to sense my own presence, I guess.'

'Mhmm, so you wanted to reach out and let him know you were there in a sup-portive kind of way?'

'But I didn't say that, I mean, I'd already said something about him taking his time, I only wanted to understand. But I could have said, "I'm here for you when you feel able to talk about it", but I introduced the scariness.'

'Did he look scared?'

'No, anxious, intense.' Charlotte tried to think back to the moment that it had happened. 'Like he was fighting with himself, or maybe that's a projection because I know what he talked about afterwards. No, he looked as though he was struggling with something.'

'So Ali looks as though he is struggling with something, and you seek to reach out to him with an emphasis on it being scary, yes?'

Charlotte took a deep breath and sighed. 'Yes, I did. I didn't respond to the strug-gle, I noticed it but it got lost. And I brought in the scariness. And it was then that he began to knock his clenched fists together,' she demonstrated the move-ment, 'faster and faster'. We didn't really explore that, in fact I applied pre-therapy responses as it really felt as though he had moved out of psychological contact. When he came back in contact with me he talked about there being this voice in his head. He seemed to be trying to focus himself. But where did the idea of scariness come from?'

'What do you think, given what we were saying earlier?'

'Maybe part of me feels scared witnessing the kind of struggle that was happening for Ali. Maybe something about him made some part of me feel scared, but my reality in that moment was not one of feeling scared myself.'

'OK, so the question is then whether within you there is a part of you that carries scariness in association with this kind of experience, but you are not in conscious touch with that part, but it can communicate.'

However much training, therapy and personal development work undertaken, there remains the possibility that there will be areas within that have not been fully explored. The counsellor, however experienced, has to remain open to the possibility that they will uncover aspects of themselves which were previously unknown. It is for this reason that becoming a person-centred counsellor is to enter on a journey of life-long learning.

Charlotte frowned as she thought about this, and its meaning. She could feel herself struggling with the idea that there were parts of herself that she was not aware of. She must be aware of them. She was an experienced therapist, but did she really know herself? Were there still blind spots. She didn't like the idea. She didn't like the idea of not having the word 'control' came to mind. Not having control, not knowing what was going on inside herself. That felt scary. The notion of scariness wasn't a thought, it was a feeling that was suddenly very present for her.

Matt noted a change in Charlotte's expression. It suddenly looked very serious. He responded to what he saw. 'The way you look appears to me very serious.'

Charlotte felt slightly spaced out in herself. Something was happening inside her. She knew she had to explore it. 'I'm in a place where the thought of not knowing what is within my structure of self, and of therefore not feeling in control of who I am, well, that feels scary.' She looked across at Matt. 'Scary.'

Matt nodded. 'Mhmm. Scary to not feel in control.'

'For me, for me it's scary. May not be for someone else, though it probably should be, but for me it is scary. I have to own that and be aware that I actually feel that quite intensely. And yet it isn't something I feel generally. I ...' She thought back to that last session with Ali. 'Is it around his mental state, the fact that he has been diagnosed as being psychotic? Is that heightening my sense of no control and triggering my own anxiety? Is it anxiety?' She thought about it, allowing the feeling to become more present. It was in her solar plexus region, a deep sense of unease. She nodded. 'I am uneasy about this.' Charlotte paused again. 'It feels like a kind of edge.'

'Edge?'

Charlotte nodded again but remained deep in thought. What did she mean by 'edge'? 'Like being close to something other, something unknown, something . . . , yes, something' She couldn't find a word that seemed to fit. Alien – no, that didn't sound right. Edge, edge of what?

Matt noted the frown still on Charlotte's face. He knew she was trying to work it through for herself. He respected her own internal processing and waited for when she was ready to communicate whatever it was she was experiencing.

'Edge. What do we mean by an edge? It's a boundary, a point or a line at which something ends and something else begins, perhaps? Or maybe it's like the edge on an horizon, it isn't that something ends and something else begins, it's the same continuum but it's out of sight. Out of sight . . . So.' Charlotte paused, trying to draw her thoughts together. 'So, something about being aware of an edge brings a sense of scariness to me.' She thought again as a fresh train of thought emerged for her. Edges and boundaries. She felt she was a well-boundaried therapist. She kept her boundaries, it was a professional require-ment. She took a deep breath. 'Sorry, I'm in here processing. It's just triggered another line of thought for me.'

'Go on.'

'Well, edges are boundaries, and I feel I do keep boundaries, that it's one of my strengths.'

'Mhmm, I would agree with that, Charlotte.'

'And I see it as a professional requirement, something that I do and maintain as part of my professionalism.'

'Sure, your clear boundaries and you being professional.'

'Yes, but what if they aren't?'

It was Matt's turn to frown. 'Sorry, you mean, "what if your boundaries are unprofessional?".' He was unclear.

'No, the boundaries are professional but the motivation for having them isn't.'

'You mean your reasons for having boundaries are for reasons other than profes-sionalism?'

Charlotte nodded. 'Supposing my boundaries are not being driven by professional need but by personal need? I need clear boundaries. I need to know where the edge is so I can keep away from it because to get too close, or to even think too much about what's over the edge, as it were, is too scary.'

Matt breathed deeply and sat back slightly. 'Right, I've got you. So you wonder whether your clear boundariedness is being motivated by your own personal feelings about being too close to an edge.'

'And the risk of not being in control that is associated with going over that edge, or beyond it. The idea of an horizon was one of the things that came to mind just now, of how an horizon appears to be an edge and yet it isn't really. But the thought that it is makes it something that can provoke anxiety if you thought you might have to go close to that edge.'

'Probably stopped ancient mariners exploring too far in case they fell off the world.'

'Right. So does my concept of an edge, and this feels scary, but a different kind of scary. Does my concept of an edge in terms of human experience stop me from exploring?'

'Your edge, or the client's edge?'

Charlotte's immediate reaction was her client's edge, but she hesitated. No, it wasn't just the client's edge, it was her's as well. 'Both, either. Any edge. Getting close to an edge in my own understanding or knowledge, or a client being on an edge that seemed to be getting close to my experiential horizon maybe? I haven't thought this through. But there is something about edges being scary, and coming back to what I was saying, does my being good with boundaries emerge out of my anxiety around edges more than my professionalism?' Another deep breath. She looked searchingly towards Matt. 'It's a big one, isn't it?'

Matt nodded, and was aware that he hadn't really had this discussion before, either about himself or with supervisees. And yet it seemed suddenly to have such relevance as an issue.

'It feels big, and makes me think of me as well. So, there is something then, perhaps, about what happened with Ali in that session that took you to a sense of an edge, provoked somewhere, somehow, a sense of scariness which, at the time, you were not conscious of, but which contributed to you responding to him in such a way that you highlighted the idea that it must be scary for him even though he was actually looking serious and concentrated?'

Charlotte listened and reflected on what Matt was saying. It sounded like a really good summary. She wished she could be clear like that, sometimes. 'And in a way, well, the session moved on and we got into exploring what the voices said, and he was able to identify a part in himself which he called "jailbreak" which is about wanting to get away, break free.'

Matt nodded, aware that Charlotte had moved on whilst he felt that there was a need to stay further with the topic of edges and boundaries, scariness and anxiety. The incident in the session may not have been in any way damaging for the therapeutic process, but it had opened up an area requiring exploration for Charlotte.

'OK, so the session moved on. But I'm still with the notion of the edge provoking unexperienced but communicated scariness, if that was what was happening for you.'

Charlotte put her hand across her mouth, resting her elbow on her other hand as she thought about it. She held her breath as she reflected further. 'Maybe I'm not as comfortable working with a client presenting with the kind of experiences that Ali has as I thought I was. Deep down, maybe I am uneasy about working at ...' She pondered a phrase that came to mind, '... working at the psychotic edge. And having said that, you know, I want to unsay it because I don't, fundamentally, believe in that diagnosis in the sense that it's a social construct, like the horizon. No, well, the horizon's not a social construct but the meaning we attribute to it is.'

'Something about the meaning of "psychotic edge"?'

'If human beings, well ...' Charlotte couldn't quite think of how to say what she was thinking. Her sense was that people extended beyond their normal selves. She didn't like the word normal, another social construct. 'Acceptable and unacceptable thinking, there's a boundary. It's OK to have a feeling to act in a particular way, a kind of hunch, but when it's a voice in your head telling you to do it then it becomes unacceptable. But it's a continuum, that's how I see it. So, I may have a kind of hunch or an urge to, say, go to the beach. That's fine. Quite normal and acceptable. But it could be that there is something else more urgent to attend to, but I still act on the inner urge. Well, still acceptable, but maybe it could be questioned. Perhaps I am meeting a stronger need to get away from something, either way I am now acting in a manner that is perhaps out of phase with what needs to be done. But generally that's still OK. But if I have a voice telling me to go to the beach, or commanding me to go, when there is something else to attend to, what then? It begins to become more unacceptable.'

'To whom?'

'I guess others who may be thinking, "why did she do that when she needed to do this?".'

'OK.'

'And then the next extreme is the voice telling someone to do something that is harmful to themselves or others. Then it becomes a mental health problem, at least, that's how it seems to be. It's OK to have voices, but not if they tell you to act bizarrely or in an antisocial way.'

'So it is the content of the voice and the nature of the behaviour that defines whether the person is on a psychotic edge.'

'But it could be normal to them. I guess the extreme situations where people are at risk to themselves or others, yes, that needs addressing for reasons of safety and risk. But if there is no risk or safety issue, but say someone hears a voice telling them, I don't know, to spend their life feeding pigeons because that is what God wants them to do, and they hear God's voice very clearly. It's a daft example, but no one is being harmed. Is that psychotic? Or is that someone who likes birds, wants to feel good about caring for birds, and they have created a way of giving themselves permission to do this?'

'Mhmm, not sure where you are going, but OK.'

'Neither am I, but it is something about, for me, the idea of a psychotic edge. Part of me feels that it is a construct, it's inconsistent, and yet there are severely disturbed people who clearly live beyond my horizon, who experience things which trigger behaviours that are outside my knowledge and understanding. People who, if you like, are over my edge.'

Matt smiled. 'And that's the crucial factor. Who's edge? Who defines the edge? For you, working with a client, it is your edge that matters in terms of your ability to be a companion with that client, yes? That's what we have to deal with. Yes, the broader debate remains, but in therapy, as a counsellor, can you define your edge and can you work with people who are close to or over that edge?'

'And that's about professional and personal competence?'

'Yes.'

Charlotte suddenly felt clearer. 'This is really helping. Getting this out, exploring, just going through this process. I've not talked like this before, it is helpful. I have to define my edge. And in that session Ali was on that edge and maybe over it, and so I have to extend my horizon.'

'He's helping you do that, in a way. The question is when he invites you into his world, beyond your horizon, can you take that journey with him and still be able to get back into the world this side of it?'

Charlotte nodded, but somehow the idea didn't feel as scary as it had done before. Now she had a metaphor, no, it was more than a metaphor, a framework within which to operate. She could maintain professional boundaries for professional reasons, but her own psychological and emotional boundaries needed to be more open, and she needed to be at ease with that.

'I really appreciate this. This discussion and exploration, well, it has itself extended my horizon, it really has. And it all happened through this process. My calmness in the session may have been sort of false, but my anxiety emerged through my reference to it being scary for Ali. Perhaps I can now experience more of a genuine calmness and also a clearer connection with my own sense of my scariness of sailing close to the edge. I'm back to the ancient explorers wondering if they'd fall off the edge of the world.'

'And it was a reasonable view in the context of the knowledge and understanding of the time.'

'I wonder how our current ideas around mental health will be viewed in the future when we travel beyond our current horizon in our treatment and understanding of mental health problems, and, of course, substance use?'

The focus of the supervision moved on to another client. For both Charlotte and Matt it had been a valuable dialogue, extending themselves as they grappled with the notion of working with clients who exist close to an edge, and the impact that this can have on the counsellor.

Points for discussion

- How do you feel about Ali? What thoughts and reactions are present for you?
- The notion of having to work with clients who exist beyond your own horizon – what does this bring up for you?
- Do you feel the content of the supervision session was appropriate?
- How can the actualising tendency be most effectively facilitated when working with a client experiencing significant mental disturbance? Would you have responded differently at any point to anything that Charlotte introduced into the supervision session?
- How much should theoretical speculation form part of supervision?
- Write supervision notes for this session.

CHAPTER 11

Supervising the counselling of a recovering drug user*

Drug use is widespread and, worryingly, is being developed at earlier ages and with an increasing tendency towards 'polydrug' use – using more than one drug. Counsellors need to be prepared to work with people who are using, or who have had a history of using, substances. It brings up a range of issues rooted in stereotypical thinking about people who use drugs. Yet the counsellor needs to address their own preconceptions and any judgementalism that may be present for them if they are truly to be able to offer a genuine therapeutic relationship with a member of this client group.

Dan is on a methadone prescription (methadone is a medically prescribed pharmaceutical product that to some degree mimics the opiate effects of heroin). He has had a history of heroin use. Many heroin users are prescribed methadone as part of their treatment programme to help them keep away from street drugs and damaging injecting practices, and to provide some stability which, in turn, can offer an opportunity for counselling to help them make sense of themselves and their lives, work on underlying issues, and maybe begin to reduce their dependence on their substance use.

Dan has referred himself to a local drug agency where Jeannie is a volunteer counsellor. She has a number of years experience and finds it very rewarding. Dan has been offered eight sessions and he has attended seven. The one he missed was because he was in hospital – bad reaction to injecting. He has used a range of substances, starting in childhood sniffing glue. Dan's brother was killed in the army and his father was a heavy and at times violent drinker. Like many drug users in treatment, he had used other substances whilst also taking his prescribed methadone. He wants to change but it is a struggle. His girlfriend, Gemma, is supportive although it has not been an easy relationship.

There are two supervision sessions in this chapter. The first follows the counselling session in which Dan discloses how he had witnessed his best friend, Billy, die in front of him as a child; the result of sniffing aerosols. A lot of emotion was

---

*Taken from *Counselling a Recovering Drug User: a person-centred dialogue* (2003) by Richard Bryant-Jefferies. Radcliffe Medical Press, Oxford.

released as he connected with the painful feelings associated with the experience and Jeannie offered him her calm and non-judgemental presence as he described how they had at first laughed at Billy, thinking he was fooling around, before realising that he was unable to breathe and dying in front of their eyes.

The second supervision session contains an exploration of Dan's process of engaging with and defining different 'parts' of himself, and includes references to Mearns' theory regarding 'configurations within self' (Mearns and Thorne, 1999, 2000). Jeannie, Dan's counsellor, is supervised privately by Max.

Supervision session 1

Supervisor: Max

Supervisee/Counsellor: Jeannie

Client: Dan

'I need some time today on Dan, my new client at the agency that I spoke about a month ago.'

'Yes, I remember, on methadone and trying to move on, but with a long history of using all kinds of substances, but generally suppressants.'

'Yes. Well, a lot has happened, Max, and it is hard to know where to begin.' Jeannie stopped and thought about it. She continued. 'In a way I really want to talk about me because I experienced a really powerful reaction to him after the last session, though I feel I need to explain what has been happening to put my reaction in context.'

Max nodded. 'So, major concern about a reaction that you had but it sounds like a lot has been going on.'

'That's an understatement!'

'Tell me about it.'

'Well, a few sessions back, probably the first after I saw you, he had a panic attack, and that was somewhat unnerving, and I remember a sense that somehow his body was trying to tell me something? Seemed like he was maybe getting close to something inside himself but was choosing not to talk about it, but his body was communicating huge amounts of anxiety. I highlighted it, offering him the opportunity to pick up on it, but he didn't. He wanted to emphasise his need to move on. I was left wondering if I should have stayed with a focus on his bodily reaction a bit more, try to help him explore it, but I also know that I respect his choice to focus on what was important to him, and maybe at that time he just wasn't in a place to do that. I now believe that this was the case, and it was right to let it go and stay with him.'

The person-centred counsellor would expect to stay with the client, only voicing their own feelings, reactions, thoughts or perceptions where they were strong and persistent, and were genuinely felt to be emerging as a result of their contact and communication with the client. It is possible for a client to consistently speak in ways that are incongruent to their body language, for instance someone describing themselves as feeling relaxed or OK about something when in fact their body is strained and they are constantly moving their hands in an anxious and distracting manner.

In such instances, the client is communicating two experiences, and the person-centred counsellor can helpfully empathise with both, not necessarily pointing out the contradiction which would be an interpretation, but simply letting the client know what they are experiencing as being communicated to them. The client is thereby offered the opportunity to clarify their body language if they wish to. Either way, that part of them which is driving the body has an opportunity to feel heard and may then find its voice if the client's process allows it.

'Was this something you wondered at the time, or in hindsight? I am curious as to whether your experience was, if you like, in real time, in the moment of connecting with the client, or if it was in retrospect?'

'I thought about it at the time, but it didn't feel a big issue. I guess it was later that I began to wonder. He moved on to talk about something else, his girlfriend I think, I'm not sure now, and I guess it was after the session that I was aware that actually something that had seemed quite major had occurred but then kind of left behind somehow. But things happened which provoked, maybe that's not the right word, but certainly encouraged Dan to disclose what I think may well have been behind the panic attack, although it is speculation.'

Max was intrigued. He was aware Jeannie was talking a lot but he wasn't really getting many facts. He wondered if it was a parallel process. He voiced his wondering.

Parallel processing is where a feature of the client's experiencing is played out within someone else. In this instance it is the content of what Jeannie is saying that Max is wondering if it is a parallel process, reflecting something of the way that the client presents his story. It can be useful to identify and work with as it can often shed light on what may be present for the client. It is often indicative of a powerful dynamic being present within the client. Working with it in supervision can highlight how much the counsellor has been drawn into this dynamic which could impact on their ability to be congruent or block accurate empathy.

'I sort of have this feeling that you are saying a lot but not telling me much. Lots of references to things happening but not sure what they are yet, and I know you are getting to them, but I am wondering if this process is actually reflecting something about the client, or your relationship with the client.'

Jeannie thought about it. Lots of words but not much information. She reflected back on what she knew about Dan. She knew of some key events in his life, and she had experienced being with him whilst he experienced the deep hurt, the sense of guilt, of anxiety that had emerged in the sessions. Max was right. She knew a little, but there were big gaps. She knew nothing about his prison experiences, of his early childhood, well not much about his teenage years either, other than references to his drug use and obviously the impact of the death of his brother. But yes, Max was right, she didn't know much although she felt she had experienced such a lot with Dan. Curious, she thought.

What Jeannie has recognised is important. She has a concept of having connected with Dan, she has a lot to talk about, and yet there is so much of him that she is unaware of. Maintaining her false sense of their relationship might block exploring the areas that are currently invisible to her. She needs to be open to an awareness that there is more, much more, to Dan than that which she has experienced so far.

'There are big gaps, a lot I don't know about him, and yet at another level, at a feeling level, I really do feel I have connected deeply with him and do know him. But there is a kind of split here somehow. Or is it just that we have only had eight, no seven sessions, he didn't attend one, and there was the session he was stoned. But no, it's like I have kinds of snapshots of events, pretty traumatic events, but specific events in his life.' She paused and thought about it some more. 'Maybe that's how it is for Dan. Maybe he isn't connected with everything that has happened, bits forgotten, and he is giving me himself in the way that he experiences himself. I hadn't thought of that. But it makes sense the more I think about it.'

Max wanted to encourage Jeannie to think about the implications this had for their relationship and the work they were doing. He asked about this.

Jeannie felt that maybe Dan would begin to make connections, in a sense begin to perhaps join up the events and how they impacted on him. 'He's wary, isn't he?', she suddenly said. 'He is taking time to trust me, telling me what he feels able to allow me to hear, at least that's maybe how it started. I think that is changing. I think, I know, he is now telling me things that he knows he has to say, that he needs to say. He's not controlling his disclosures in the same way – and control must be big for him – because, well, let me explain what happened. He dropped his methadone over a weekend after drinking too much the night before, and ended up injecting heroin, for what seemed like at least a couple of days, tried to avoid telling his girlfriend, but ended up developing a deep-vein thrombosis in his leg – he'd injected in the groin. Put him in hospital. And he also had a really deep experience as well, a kind of vision of a mountain he was being drawn towards, happened in the session, then he dreamt about it but it was different and it made him realise he had something he needed to talk about. We had a couple of really deep connections, felt spiritual. But anyway, what came out of the last session was that when he was about nine his best friend died in front of him, respiratory failure as a result of sniffing some kind of solvent, and he blames himself for his death – he had got the stuff that Billy, his friend, had sniffed. Watched him go blue and die in front of him. Has carried it around in his head for years, telling no one what he felt, and clearly has used substances to try and blot it out. And I think he has been punishing himself as well, maybe that's part of his drug use, and getting into prison, I don't know, I may be running ahead on that. He hasn't made that connection and I'm not going to suggest it.'

Counselling, and particularly person-centred counselling, is not about making connections for the client. It is better for them to be supported through their own process of making sense of themselves. The offering of the core conditions facilitates this process, by offering an atmosphere in which the client gradually feels freer to move around within themselves, where their conditions of worth are less actively dominant and they can begin to take often tentative steps towards developing a fresh perspective on themselves and their past and present experiences.

'No, that would certainly be outside of a person-centred way of working. He has to be allowed to move at his own pace, make his own connections when he is able to.'

Jeannie nodded. 'Yeah, I know.' She yawned. 'Gee, I feel tired all of a sudden.' She yawned again. 'Oh, sorry, it's just come over me.' She yawned again, and again, and again. 'My eyes suddenly feel really gritty.'

'Really gritty.'

Jeannie nodded.

'Something's leaving or making you really tired, yes, so what were we saying, or were you thinking or experiencing just before it started?'

Perhaps Max should have simply stayed with Jeannie in her tiredness rather than directing her back to what they had been discussing. This would have arguably been a more person-centred response.

'I made the comment about him maybe punishing himself.' As she said it she felt another yawn coming on, a really big one, forcing her to really open her mouth wide. 'Oh dear.' She promptly yawned again, feeling the back of her jaw straining as she did so. 'God, I'm so tired.'

'Tired of?'

'I don't know. I know I'm the one that's tired, but am I tired of Dan? I don't think
so. I feel really touched by what he has gone through, and I really am wanting
to be there for him and help him make sense of it all and move on. I feel, I was
feeling, quite energised, although quite sad as well when I think about his early
life. But I . . . I don't feel tired of him, and yet . . . , oh here I go again.' Another
big yawn, and another. 'Are you feeling tired?'

Max wasn't. 'No, and your yawns don't seem to be provoking yawns in me, which
is unusual because they often seem strangely contagious.'

'So it has to be me, but I'm not aware of anything I'm tired of. Could I be tuning
into Dan? What was it we were saying, about . . .' She thought back, 'yes, I was
speculating about whether he was . . .' another yawn, 'punishing himself,'
another yawn. 'That's it. He is tired of punishing himself, or maybe part of
him,' another yawn, 'is tired of,' another yawn, 'punishing himself. Maybe
that's why he told me about Billy's death, maybe he's tired of carrying around
the memory and the guilt, even though he also told me that he would never
forget it and would blame himself for the rest of his life, at least, I think that's
what he said. Something like that, anyway.'

Jeannie closed her eyes it felt good. 'He's at risk, Max, he may not simply be tired of
carrying his feelings and memories, maybe he wants to close his eyes to it all,
and the way he has always done that is with drugs. Oh shit, I know this may
seem crazy, but I think he's at risk of another lapse, even though he wants to
get free of the drugs and the alcohol – yes, he said he stopped sniffing after Billy
died, but began using alcohol to help him forget it, blot it out, dull his feelings.
So alcohol he associates with dealing with Billy, whilst heroin is associated
with dealing with his brother, at least injecting heroin, he was already smoking
it. I think that's how it was. Again, bits.'

Max was stuck with something and unclear. He felt he needed clarity. 'I feel a bit
lost on why you are saying you feel he is at risk.'

'The sense that if he is tired of it all but cannot get rid of it by talking it through
and out, by releasing feelings, he may go back to substances. But that's
obvious. I think I'm losing the plot here, getting myself tangled up.'

'It is complex, Jeannie, lots of threads and at the moment it seems that Dan hasn't
got them connected.'

'I guess I'm struggling with it too.'

Max was suddenly aware that Jeannie hadn't yawned for a while. 'You're not
yawning.'

'No, I'm not am I. So what happened here? Recognising the complexity, the risk?
Talking has somehow released the tiredness? Is that what it's telling me, that
talking it through may, for Dan, release his being tired of it all?'

'Speculation, but maybe. Something has happened. How are you feeling?'

'Different. Lighter. Less burdened somehow.' She shook her head. 'What was that
all about?'

'I don't know, but it seems to have shifted something for you. Anything else
changed?'

Jeannie did a reality check on herself. She brought Dan back to mind, and watched her reactions as she did so. She felt less anxious. She felt a kind of OKness about him, as if she knew all would be OK. Was she fooling herself, avoiding something, or was this genuine? It felt genuine. She described it to Max. 'I feel less burdened and have a sense that all will be OK with Dan. I can't give you a reason, but that's how I feel.'

'Less burdened by Dan?'

Jeannie smiled. 'Yes, that's got to be part of it, hasn't it, I had such a strong reaction after the last session when I got back to my car to drive home, a wave of sadness hit me. Maybe I've been carrying Dan around with me more than I realised. Maybe he has affected me without me fully realising it. Not that I don't want to be affected, I do. I have to be to be effective, but maybe I need to talk things through more often, maybe I need supervision more regularly on this client.'

'Try to stop it building up?'

'Maybe. I'm concerned that if I am overloading without realising it then it may start to affect my ability to be with and stay with him. Stay with him. Shit. I lost him at a really critical moment, when he said about believing he killed Billy, I lost him. I felt my own sadness for him and ..., oh yes, here we go, ended up speculating in my own mind about how he may be punishing himself. And that's what set me off here being tired, wasn't it? OK, so, something is happening in me making it difficult to hear Dan and it seems to be linked to profound sadness and the notion of self-punishment, and being tired of it all.'

Working with people who have been deeply affected by traumatic experiences, or who carry strong, emotional content, even when it is bottled up and not expressed, can threaten to overwhelm the person-centred counsellor who is seeking to maintain openness to their client and to their own experiencing. The need not only for regular, supportive supervision but also other recreational experiences is vitally important to enable the counsellor to unwind, and dissipate emotional knots that can develop and block empathic sensitivity.

'So you lost your empathic rapport, unable to stay with him because of sadness and feeling tired?'

'No, I wasn't feeling tired at that time, just sadness and then thoughts about punishment. Let me think about this for a moment, and try and get a sense of what is present for me now.' Jeannie tried to reconnect with that sadness, she brought back to her mind that image of Dan as a boy, of the terror and the guilt, of having no one to talk to, of being huddled together with his brother and sister at home ... She began to feel her eyes watering, and tears trickling down her cheeks. She felt a lump in her throat. She allowed the feelings to flow through her and the tears continued to trickle from her eyes. She screwed her eyes up as another wave of sadness and emotion hit her. It passed, and she felt relief. She swallowed and took a deep breath. 'I still don't know what this is about, other than maybe I simply feel affected by his story, it just feels so enormous, so overwhelming. I just can't really get a sense of exactly what it must be, or have been, like. Yeah, I cry tears for him, and I am glad to have released them. It isn't bringing anything personal up for me, I think I'm just very touched by his life, his struggle, and the feelings he has kept to himself for so many years.'

'Yeah, he really has released sadness in you.'

'Yeah, and it's good to let it go. I needed to. I need to watch I don't build up again.' Jeannie took another deep breath. 'OK, I think that's what I needed.' She glanced up at the clock. 'That time already. OK, I think I'm clear for now, and, look, can I call you if I sense it's building up, or if I lose contact with Dan again in the session? I think I need to really have the availability of extra support here if I need it, though maybe I have done enough for now.'

Max agreed to this, and they decided that Jeannie could call him if she needed to talk anything through, and if he couldn't talk at the time then they'd arrange a time for a 'phone call ... That felt good, Jeannie thought, as she prepared to leave and head back home. She was so glad she worked in a profession in which supervision of this nature was part of the professional requirement to practice. Time to explore personal reactions was so precious, so important, both for her own wellbeing and to ensure that she was more likely to keep in contact with her clients during sessions. She didn't want to lose Dan again at a critical moment, he deserved better than that.

Supervision session 2

Jeannie has been discussing the idea of 'configurations within self', the notion that the structure of self is formed of 'parts', each having particular associated thoughts, feelings and behaviours which cluster and can become quite differentiated and individual in their expression. The first part of the following supervision session explores this theory.

'So, you have found yourself working with configuration of self with Dan?'

'Yes, and it has been very interesting and I have been surprised by the strength of identity that they have, and it left me wondering what that was about.'

'How do you mean?'

'Well, it was in that session where he really seemed to be talking from two of the configurations, "the addict" and what came to be known as "little boy blue". I was left wondering after the session whether the chemical impact of drug use might somehow affect the potency and individuality of configuration.'

'Interesting thought, and probably not an area that there has been much investigation into.'

'It seemed that the parts of Dan that emerged had something about them that made them seem more like dissociated parts, and yet they weren't, as far as I know, developed out of traumatic experience such as sexual abuse, at least, I assume not. Of course, that could still be a factor that Dan is quite unaware of or not voicing, but I don't think so. But I could be wrong.'

'So maybe it would be helpful to contrast configurations within the self and dissociated process. Let's see what's written.'

Max reached over to the book shelf and took down a copy of *Person-Centred Therapy Today* (Mearns and Thorne, 2000) 'Mearns writes of configurations which are established around introjects, dissonant self-dissonant self-experiences and he highlights the presence of what he terms "growth and not-for-growth" configurations' (pp. 108–16). And, yes, here we are, the chapter by Margaret Warner. She writes that 'dissociated experiences . . . are a great deal more personified than ordinary mood states or even "configurations"' (p. 162). And here, 'dissociated process seems to arise almost exclusively as a response to early childhood trauma' (p. 158). She goes on to say that these dissociated parts 'seem to emerge when trauma memories are pressing to the surface' (p. 163).

'OK, but what differentiates them?'

'OK, so what about contrasting the two concepts? Yes, here we are,' Max continued reading from Mearns. 'One key difference is linked to the "protective" function of the parts, leading, in dissociated process to some of the "parts" becoming dissociated from each other to the extent that there is a loss of awareness between parts' (p. 108). Max read also 'it is important to note that while the notion of "configurations" within the self may bear some similarities with dissociated process, it is not on a continuum with dissociative identity disorder (DID), formerly known as multiple personality disorder. In considering self in regard to "configurations", we are embracing "normal" dimensions of personality integration' (p. 108).

'OK, so no continuum, we are talking about different developments within the self.'

'Right.' Mearns goes on to refer to Ross (1999) writing about 'pluralism within the self not being on a "dissociative continuum" with DID', and then suggests that there is a 'qualitative difference in the *personification* of the parts – the parts may even have "people" names rather than descriptive titles which is more common in configurations and that there is a much more profound *separateness* between the parts' (p. 108). 'So, the personification and separateness of the parts seem to be important factors.'

'And my understanding is that with dissociative process, "parts" can even be unaware of each other.' Jeannie felt she was getting some clarity now on an area that had often been a bit of a mystery.

'Yes, so it seems a matter of degree but with a very definite need to bear in mind the origin, and the important factor of the experience of traumatic child abuse.'

'Mhmm. So, dissociated states are likely to emerge out of early childhood traumatic experiencing, in particular sexual abuse, whereas configurations are a normal development, simply the parts that make up the self and which we develop and live out of or through as we move through different experiences in life.' Jeannie thought back to her sessions. 'I'm not sure what we have here. I mean, they seemed like configurations although there has been trauma involved, as I mentioned earlier, yet there does seem to be a distinctiveness. The violence at home may not have triggered a dissociative process but then there may be factors and experiences that Dan has not talked about.'

'Mhmm.'

'Plus, of course, there is the factor of the chemical use from an early age and what impact that might have had on brain chemistry, neural pathway development and Dan's own direct experience of himself, and therefore on his own processing of parts of himself that had emerged or were to emerge later. Could configurations get more fixed through the kinds of chemicals Dan was using? I don't know. I do just wonder.'

'Something to look up and check out.' He paused. 'Perhaps what is important here is the work you are doing in allowing Dan to appreciate the different parts of himself, whatever their origin, and to provide a safe environment for this to occur.'

'I think safety is a big issue. There is a lot of vulnerability and sensitivity. Dan is showing aspects of himself to me, and in a sense realising them about himself as well. I don't want to get too tangled up in complexity and lose my simplicity of being a companion to his journey into himself.'

Max nodded.

'Whatever the origin of the parts that are present for Dan, he needs a place to bring them – should I say be them – in which all feel equally accepted, yes?'

'Yes.'

'And he must be sufficiently trusting of me and our relationship for him to reveal them, or for them to reveal themselves.'

'Mhmm.'

'And we know that more parts may emerge, I mean, the number of configurations that could have been developed in response to introjects could be large. And if there is dissociative process at work, there may be parts that have yet to appear of which Dan, and the other parts, are quite unaware of.'

'So Dan really needs you to be warmly accepting of him, all of him, to be authentically present and empathically accurate, to offer an opportunity for him to be fully present, or should I say all of him to become fully present.'

'Yes. And I really need to trust his process, don't I? I mean, I know that, but I *really* have to be there.'

'Well, yes, you are going to be operating in the dark, unsure of what might emerge at any time, having to be sensitive and responsive to whatever Dan reveals of himself.'

Such openness is extremely important as she is seeking to encourage Dan's process of being to become freer and more transparent to her. If the counsellor cannot be open and is not experienced as such by the client, then what they reveal of themselves can be blocked.

'OK. And let me just mention that Dan also moved during the counselling session towards using the metaphor of a jigsaw, with the idea of him metaphorically turning over the pieces and realising that he had to in a way decide how to fit them together and which pieces he wants as components of the person he is striving to become. And we reached the point where he could recognise that he may not know which parts to keep as he has no idea of the final picture.'

'So, pieces represent parts of Dan, and he is basically recognising the pieces and then deciding which to keep and how to fit them together.'

'Yes.'

'I think I need to think about that.' Max paused. 'But you say it seems to be helping Dan make sense of himself?'

'Yes, so I am quite happy to go with that and allow him to process it.'

'Sounds intriguing. The thought strikes me, though, that there is no finished picture, that the metaphor requires that the picture is continually evolving. Dan, or any of us, never reach a point of full functionality, or do we? Surely he will find that the picture changes as he absorbs new experiences, extracts meaning from them and his sense of self adjusts to his experiencing and the symbolisation process?'

'Hadn't thought of that. But he has realised that his choices and decisions now govern what or how he finally emerges from his process and I think that recognition has had a profound impact on him.'

'That he is responsible for his own process and outcome?'

'Yes, particularly as responsibility hasn't been a quality hugely in evidence, at least, that's what he has indicated.'

'You really are connecting with Dan and working across so much of his sense of self.'

'He has given me a lot since I last saw you, and some very painful and difficult experiences too. Seeing his best friend die in front of him, what a traumatic experience that must have been. I can see that he has a long journey within therapy ahead of him and I think that the work I am doing with him may go the distance, but I may be a companion on part of his journey only.'

'I'm curious why you say that.'

Jeannie thought about it. 'I think it may be a sense of just how much work there may be to do, and maybe I'm avoiding thinking that I am taking it all on.'

'A sense of your own avoidance of so much.'

'Overwhelming. And if I feel overwhelmed at the thought, what must Dan feel? He is faced with so much change and adaptation to really move on and ensure he can achieve what he wants – a sustainable drug-free life. I really do admire him. He seems to be persevering so far. He's a regular attendee, only missed that session when he had lapsed.'

'Yes, he is showing real commitment, and you feel a sense of admiration for him.'

'I do. He's struggling to free himself from patterns and habits.' Jeannie remembered that she had something else she wanted to check out although it seemed that it may be linked to what they had been discussing. 'There is something else that I want to raise. When I was waiting for Dan at the start of the last session, I got somewhat lost in my own thinking and as a result went out late to find him. I just started reflecting on things related to Dan and before I knew it I was ten minutes into the session. I rather feel now that it is linked to the notion of it feeling overwhelming, so many facets to think about.'

'So you found yourself immersed in thinking about Dan and it feels linked to feeling overwhelmed.'

'The sense that there is so much, so many lines of thought.'

'And the thoughts got in the way of Dan actually coming into the room.' Max knew he was being a little provocative, but he wanted to explore this further.

Jeannie nodded. 'Yes. Yes, stopped him coming in the room, it did, didn't it. Was I protecting myself in some way, I wonder? Last time we talked about me feeling overloaded and what effect that could be having. I guess it is still happening, but has come out in a different way. I'm not aware of having lost focus in the sessions, though. And I'm not feeling tired either talking about him, so something has shifted there as well. But I have to keep my discipline on this.'

'I think it is easy to get caught up in the complexities of theory here, and in a sense we kind of paralleled that earlier. I mean, I don't often get a book off the shelf and start quoting it at supervisees! So, something stirred me up as well, left me feeling a need to do that. Just seems to be something around the complexity of Dan and maybe we are both struggling in different ways to feel, I don't know, on top of it? Does that sound right?'

Jeannie wasn't sure. 'For me it is about feeling able to be open and fully present.'

'Of course, so why do I go and say "on top of it"?'

'Want to explore it? May have some relevance here.' Jeannie was aware of a kind of role reversal but she felt OK with that. It had sounded odd what Max had said and maybe it did have some connection to Dan's complexity.

Roles are reversed and Jeannie has encouraged Max to explore his experience and reaction. After all, they are forming a therapeutic relationship, albeit supervisory in nature, and when the supervisor experiences something relevant it can be usefully explored then and there in the session. In the final analysis, supervisor and supervisee are co-professionals, working together collaboratively.

Max nodded. 'I suppose it is about getting a handle on what is going on, and somehow as I say that I immediately hear a little voice inside myself saying, "so you're not trusting the process". And maybe that's it, I am not trusting the process and perhaps that is about the chemical impact of the drugs. I know that the actualising tendency will continue to operate, but I just have a sense that there is a chemical barrier and it's making it difficult for me to get a grip on the situation. It feels foggy.'

Jeannie broke out in goosebumps. 'When I saw you last, had I mentioned the green fog?'

'I don't recall that.'

'No, of course, it was the session before last. Dan talked about being in a green fog, holding him back, making him feel stuck, yet keeping him from knowing what was outside of it. Well he mentioned that "the addict" made him drink it, and it became clear that it had to be the methadone.'

'I'm getting affected by the fogginess? Struggling to get a grip, to, as I said, "get on top of it".'

'Makes sense?'

'Could be that I'm picking up the fogginess. Interesting that you are not tired this session, so you are maintaining clarity, but it is me that is in the fog.' Max was intrigued by all of this. He found the process of supervision fascinating and these kind of experiences always left him with a sense of wonder. He wanted to explore it more, but he knew this was Jeannie's time, and it did seem that they had made sense of it. So he decided he should take it to his supervisor and allow Jeannie the time to continue with what she wanted to bring to this supervision session.

Jeannie appreciated this and went on to talk about the hug she had given Dan and how powerful it had felt. They both acknowledged not knowing what meaning Dan ascribed to it, but that it had had a profound effect. They explored briefly the importance of physical contact being therapeutically justifiable when it proceeded out of a sense of therapeutic connectedness with the client, and the risks associated with a client misinterpreting what was intended through the physical contact.

Points for discussion

- What are the key moments during these two supervision sessions?
- What key areas do you feel a supervisor needs to be aware of when supervising the counselling of a drug user?
- Evaluate Max's responses from the perspective of person-centred theory.
- Were there areas that you felt needed further exploration and, if so, why?
- If you were Max, what might you take from these sessions to your own supervision?
- Write notes for these sessions from the standpoint of the supervisor.

Author's epilogue

Which of the supervision dialogues stand out for you, and why, and which appear to have become immediately forgettable? Which issues most affect you, and which seem irrelevant? What do you feel you have gained personally and professionally from reading to this point, and how can you apply these gains? And if you feel you have gained nothing, and the whole process of reading this book has been pointless, what can you take away from that experience?

I have enjoyed putting this book together. It has enabled me to revisit 'old friends', characters from the past which have come back to life. It has been valuable to re-write some of these sessions, adding in further comment boxes and noting where, if I had written them now, I might have changed some of the responses that the supervisors were making. In a sense the books are each written at a particular point in my development and I would hope that, were I to attempt to re-write any of them at some future point, then they would take a different form, drawing from my own development and learning. Nothing is static, not when we are talking about human beings and human relationships.

I must confess to be intrigued as to whether a compilation of this kind actually works. As I write these final paragraphs I am thinking about who I should get to read it, feeling that I need someone who has not read any of the living therapy books, and maybe someone who has read them all. Will the dialogues stand alone and will they offer learning and material to reflect on? Have I given enough background from the counselling session to give the supervision sessions meaning and context? Are the supervisors sufficiently person-centred? I welcome feedback.

After writing the eight Living Therapy books so far it felt timely to attempt a focus on supervision. At times I still feel that supervision is an idea whose time is still ahead of us. It is limited to certain professions and has not been really embraced as it might be in other areas of work. I personally think person-centred supervision would be extremely valuable for overstressed and overworked managers who would benefit from time out to reflect on process and to have the space to reconnect with themselves. I am sure the same is true in many other areas of work.

I don't feel that I have much more to add. I hope the book will speak for itself. The idea of creating this book only emerged about two weeks ago, and here I am writing the epilogue. Yet it has not felt hurried.

I have referred to others who have written books, papers, chapters and paragraphs about person-centred supervision, and I hope you will want to follow these up. I like to think of a network of people all focusing their thoughts and feelings on defining and developing this practice called person-centred supervision. It feels at times like a group effort, with published ideas bouncing off people, stimulating fresh thinking.

I come back to the notion of person-centred supervision as an idea whose time has come, or is coming, I'm not sure which. But I like the thought that there is a kind of idea in the ethers that people are contributing to and shaping by their own thoughts, reflections and research. Perhaps we should think of it as the person-centred idea. It seems to me that the last decade or so has seen it receiving quite a boost and perhaps there will come a point when it will become so magnetised by the thoughts flowing into it that it will attract more and more people. Perhaps we might view it as a raincloud of knowledge, getting bigger and eventually precipitating its contents in the form of ideas into human minds.

Or am I being a little bit crazy? Well, who knows. Maybe it helps to be a little crazy. Let's be open-minded. Whatever the process, there is no doubt that the principles and values of the person-centred approach are here to stay and in so many ways they are indicative of a creative and fulfilling way forward for human beings individually and collectively. The more empathic sensitivity, unconditional positive regard and congruence expressed through genuineness, authenticity and transparency that we can muster, the greater the chance that more and more people will find their potential as persons. And then perhaps we will finally see that transformation that will enable us to truly know what being human really means in its fullest sense, and thereby claim our true heritage as 'human beings'.

I will end with a piece I wrote some years ago, drawing from Carl Rogers' thoughts about 'The Person of Tomorrow' which is taken from a section in *A Way of Being*. I wrote this short piece in the hope that it will encourage others to reflect upon aspects of Rogers' vision of the future that sometimes gets lost amongst discussions over core conditions and their sufficiency or their insufficiency to promote therapeutic movement. I wonder, and I believe it is important to take time to wonder, whether we need to look a little further; whether we need to chase a farther horizon?

Writing some years back, although I feel it remains relevant to our present time, Teilhard de Chardin suggested the following.

It has become very difficult, in the world's present state of upheaval and distraction, to form any idea of the significance of what is going on except by rising above the individual level.*

He commented that we might feel as though 'the human ship is rudderless in the storm' of ideas, passions, institutions and peoples that clash around us. As a result we can lose sight of the distant, we can lose our capacity to dream as

---

* *The Future of Man* (1964) by Teilhard de Chardin (Colling Sons and Co., London).

we float around in a sea of apparently overwhelming uncertainty. He continues as follows.

> We must rise above the storm, the chaos of surface detail, and from a higher vantage point look for the outline of some great and significant phenomenon.

Can we dare to see the present as transition, all seemingly in flux, nothing really clear or certain and yet, perhaps, somewhere deep and unseen works a purpose we have lost touch with? An inner tendency at work within us all, individually and who knows maybe collectively too, seeking to enhance our potential as sensitive, caring and more genuine human beings?

The section in *A Way of Being* that I wish to draw attention to can be found from page 350 onwards under the heading 'The qualities of the person of tomorrow' (Rogers, 1980). It seems to me that they provide us with a guiding light, shining upon us, encouraging us to take responsibility for our own way of being as persons engaging in a great process of growth within the greater human family.

Let me list these qualities and encourage you to read in Rogers' own words his interpretation and meaning of the following words.

1   Openness
2   Desire for authenticity
3   Scepticism regarding science and technology
4   Desire for wholeness
5   The wish for intimacy
6   Process persons
7   Caring
8   Attitude towards nature
9   Anti-institutional
10   The authority within
11   The unimportance of material things
12   A yearning for the spiritual.

I do not wish to quote Rogers verbatim but perhaps some of these need a little explanation in order to minimise the risk of misinterpretation. I think we all appreciate the virtue of openness and the desire for authenticity among persons. The scepticism regarding science and technology is not a 'throw the technological baby out with the scientific bath water' attitude, rather it is rooted in a deep scepticism of the use of science and technology to 'conquer' and 'dominate' nature and to use scientific power to control people. Rogers saw the need to value science where it is used to 'enhance self-awareness and control of the person by the person'.

Wholeness, intimacy and caring are words which again are reasonably self-explanatory. Process persons I find interesting in that it conjures up for me a sense of movement and of fluidity, of people who are willing to accept the uncertainty and flux of life. The attitude towards nature Rogers suggests will be present in the person of tomorrow who will be one that embraces 'a closeness to, and a caring for, elemental nature'. He saw these persons valuing alliance and coopera-tion with nature, and having ecological sensitivity and vision. Anti-institutional is about the purpose and function of institutions. There is nothing wrong with institutions, but do they really exist for the people? The person of tomorrow, Rogers foretells, will have little time for inflexible, bureaucratic institutions.

It seems clear, too, that we must learn to take greater authority from within ourselves, that we should learn to trust our own experiences and make our own judgements. And perhaps this is linked to an increasing recognition of the unim-portance of material comforts and rewards that many experience today. Finally, Rogers ends with the idea that the person of tomorrow will experience a yearning for the spiritual. This latter element seems to me crucially important as we seek to recognise the significance of therapeutic support towards what I have elsewhere referred to as transperson-centredness (Bryant-Jefferies, 1997).

Can we, do we, dare we, live to these ideals? Can we afford not to? We must each make up our own minds and make our own choices and decisions. We are all per-sons travelling along the evolutionary continuum, each seeking and receiving experiences and opportunities to grow and to enhance ourselves. We are each responsible within our own spheres of activity and influence. And in a world of global connectedness and interdependence this sphere includes not just us as individuals, but the whole human family. What does it mean to extend the person-centred vision beyond our shores and national boundaries? How should we modify our lives to ensure that we act in ways that enhance the growth potential of other people in distant lands: the street child in South America; the woman toiling in the fields of Asia; the economic refugee forced to beg on Western city streets?

We can turn away and say, 'it is not our problem'. Or, 'I am too small to make a difference'. I think these responses are rooted in ignoring that whether we like it or not we live in a global age. Person-centred living helps us to experience inner freedom to be and to become. Freedom brings responsibility. As individuals seek-ing to embrace the person-centred way of being we must, I believe, choose how we respond to human need today. For me, Rogers' 'qualities of the person of tomorrow' provide a focus towards which the actualising tendency will move us and a cutting edge within the human struggle to create a world in which we, our children and our children's children will wish to live.

References

Bozarth J (1998) *Person-Centred Therapy: a revolutionary paradigm*. PCCS Books, Ross-on-Wye.

Bozarth J and Wilkins P (eds) (2001) *Rogers' Therapeutic Conditions: evolution, theory and practice*. Volume 3: *Congruence*. PCCS Books, Ross-on-Wye.

Bryant-Jefferies R (1997) From person to transperson-centredness: a future trend. *The Person-Centred Journal*. 4(1).

Bryant-Jefferies R (2001) *Counselling the Person Beyond the Alcohol Problem*. Jessica Kingsley Publishers, London.

Bryant-Jefferies R (2003) *Counselling a Recovering Drug User: a person-centred dialogue*. Radcliffe Medical Press, Oxford.

Embleton Tudor L, Keemar K, Tudor K *et al.* (2004) *The Person-Centred Approach: a contemporary introduction*. Palgrave MacMillan, Basingstoke.

Freeth R (2004) A psychiatrist's experience of person-centred supervision. In: K Tudor and M Worrall (eds) *Freedom to Practice: person-centred approaches to supervision*. PCCS Books, Ross-on-Wye.

Gaylin N (2001) *Family, Self and Psychotherapy: a person-centred perspective*. PCCS Books, Ross-on-Wye.

Hackney H and Goodyear RK (1984) Carl Rogers' client-centred approach to supervision. In: R Levant and J Shlien (eds) *Client-Centred Therapy and the Person-Centred Approach: new directions in theory, research and practice*. Praeger, New York.

Haugh S (1998) Congruence: a confusion of language. In: T Merry (ed.) *Person-Centred Practice*. Volume 6, No. 1. PCCS Books, Ross-on-Wye.

Haugh S and Merry T (eds) (2001) *Rogers' Therapeutic Conditions: evolution, theory and practice*. Volume 2: *Empathy*. PCCS Books, Ross-on-Wye.

Kilborn M (1999) Challenge and person-centred supervision – are they compatible? *Person-Centred Practice*. 7 (2): 83–91.

Matarazzo RG and Patterson DR (1986) Methods of teaching therapeutic skill. In: SL Garfield and AE Bergin (eds) *Handbook of Psychotherapy and Behavior Change* (3e). Wiley, New York, pp. 821–43.

Mearns D (1992) On the self-concept fighting back. In: W Dryden (ed.) *Hard Earned Lessons from Counselling in Action*. Sage, London.

Mearns D (1997) *Person-Centred Counselling Training*. Sage, London.

Mearns D and Thorne B (1988) *Person-Centred Counselling in Action*. Sage, London.

Mearns D and Thorne B (1999) *Person-Centred Counselling in Action* (2e). Sage, London.

Mearns D and Thorne B (2000) *Person-Centred Therapy Today*. Sage, London.

Merry T (2001) Congruence and the supervision of client-centred therapists. In: G Wyatt (ed.) *Rogers' Therapeutic Conditions: evolution, theory and practice*. Volume 1: *Congruence*. PCCS Books, Ross-on-Wye.

Merry T (2002) *Learning and Being in Person-Centred Counselling* (2e). PCCS Books, Ross-on-Wye.

Patterson CH (1997) Client-centred supervision. In: E Watkins (ed.) *Handbook of Psychotherapy Supervision*. Wiley, New York.

Patterson CH (2000) *Understanding Psychotherapy: fifty years of client-centred theory and practice*. PCCS Books, Ross-on-Wye.

Prouty G (2002) The practice of pre-therapy. In: G Wyatt and P Sanders (eds) *Rogers' Therapeutic Conditions: evolution, theory and practice*. Volume 4: *Contact and perception*. PCCS Books, Ross-on-Wye.

Rogers CR (1957) The necessary and sufficient conditions of therapeutic personality change. *Journal of Consulting Psychology*. **21**: 95–103.

Rogers CR (1959) A theory of therapy, personality and interpersonal relationships as developed in the client-centered framework. In: S Koch (ed.) *Psychology: a study of a science*. Volume 3: *Formulations of the person and the social context*. McGraw-Hill, New York, pp. 219–35.

Rogers CR (1980) *A Way of Being*. Houghton-Mifflin, Boston, MA.

Rogers CR (1986) A client-centered/person-centered approach to therapy. In: I Kutash and A Wolfe (eds) *Psychotherapists' Casebook*. Jossey Bass, San Francisco, pp. 236–57.

Ross CA (1999) Subpersonalities and multiple personalities: a dissociative continuum. In: J Rowan and M Cooper (eds) *The Plural Self*. Sage, London, pp. 183–97.

Sommerbeck L (2003) *The Client Centred Therapist in Psychiatric Contexts*. PCCS Books, Ross-on-Wye.

Townsend I (2004) Almost nothing to do: supervision and the person-centred approach in homeopathy. In: K Tudor and M Worrall (eds) *Freedom to Practice: person-centred approaches to supervision*. PCCS Books, Ross-on-Wye.

Tudor K and Worrall M (2004) *Freedom to Practice: person-centred approaches to supervision*. PCCS Books, Ross-on-Wye.

Warner M (2002) Psychological contact, meaningful process and human nature. In: G Wyatt and P Sanders (eds) *Rogers' Therapeutic Conditions: evolution, theory and practice*. Volume 4: *Contact and perception*. PCCS Books, Ross-on-Wye, pp. 76–95.

Wheeler S (2003) *Research on Supervision of Counsellors and Psychotherapists: a systematic scoping search*. British Association for Counselling and Psychotherapy, Rugby.

Wilhelm R (1968) *I Ching or Book of Changes*. Routledge and Kegan Paul, London. Quoted in Capra F (1983) *The Turning Point*. Fontana Paperbacks, London.

Wilkins P (2003) *Person-Centred Therapy in Focus*. Sage, London.

Worrall M (2001) Supervision and empathic understanding. In: S Haugh and T Merry (eds) *Rogers' Therapeutic Conditions: evolution, theory and practice*. Volume 2: *Empathy*. PCCS Books, Ross-on-Wye.

Wyatt G (ed.) (2001) *Rogers' Therapeutic Conditions: evolution, theory and practice*. Volume 1: *Congruence*. PCCS Books, Ross-on-Wye.

Wyatt G and Sanders P (eds) (2002) *Rogers' Therapeutic Conditions: evolution, theory and practice*. Volume 4: *Contact and perception*. PCCS Books, Ross-on-Wye.

Person-centred organisations

British Association for the Person-Centred Approach (BAPCA)
Bm-BAPCA
London WC1N 3XX
Tel: 01989 770948
Email: info@bapca.org.uk
Website: www.bapca.org.uk

National association promoting the person-centred approach. Publishes the journal *Person-centred practice* and a regular Newsletter *Person-to-person*. Also maintains a directory of person-centred counsellors (including supervisors).

World Association for Person-Centered and Experiential Psychotherapy and Counselling
Email: secretariat@pce-world.org
Website: www.pce-world.org

Association for the Development of the Person-Centered Approach (ADPCA)
Email: adpca-web@signs.portents.com
Website: www.adpca.org

An international association, with members in 27 countries. For those interested in the development of client-centred therapy and the person-centred approach.

Person-Centred Therapy Scotland
Tel: 0870 7650871
Email: info@pctscotland.co.uk
Website: www.pctscotland.co.uk

An association of person-centred therapists in Scotland which offers training and networking opportunities to members with the aim of fostering high standards of professional practice.

Index